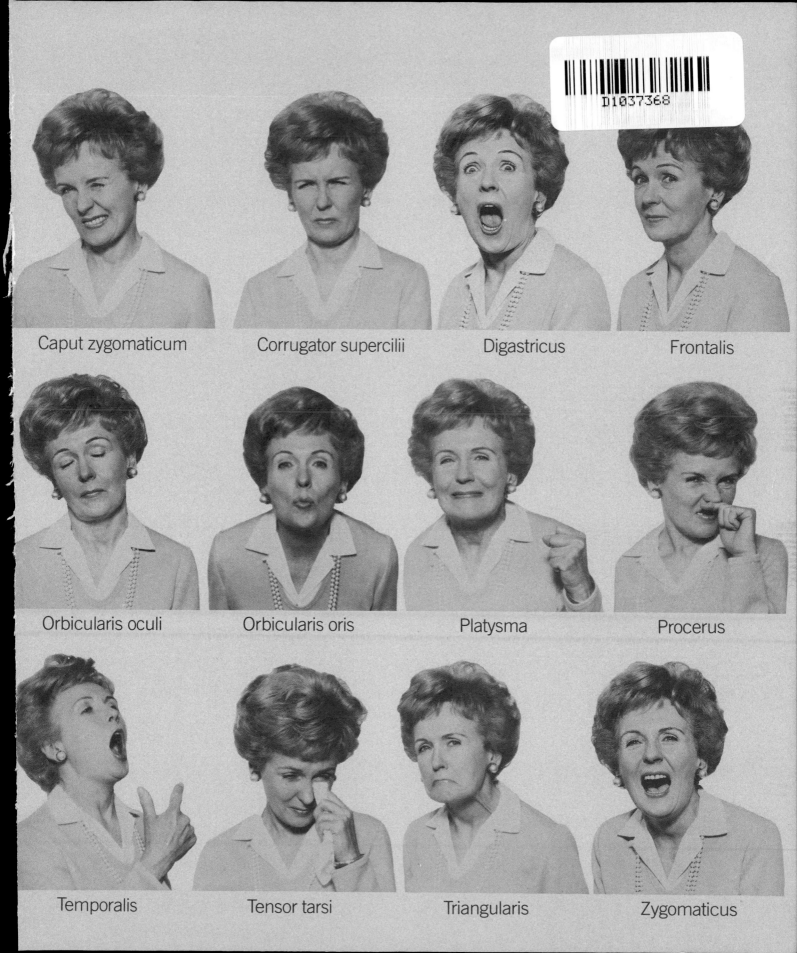

Caput zygomaticum

Corrugator supercilii

Digastricus

Frontalis

Orbicularis oculi

Orbicularis oris

Platysma

Procerus

Temporalis

Tensor tarsi

Triangularis

Zygomaticus

Miss Craig's
Face-Saving Exercises

Books by Marjorie Craig
MISS CRAIG'S 21-DAY SHAPE-UP PROGRAM FOR MEN AND WOMEN
MISS CRAIG'S FACE-SAVING EXERCISES

Miss Craig's Face-Saving Exercises

A 6-DAY PLAN WHICH TEACHES YOU HOW TO NATURALLY LIFT THE SAGGING MUSCLES OF THE FACE

All exercises demonstrated by the author, Marjorie Craig

Random House, New York

Acknowledgment is extended to Lea & Febiger for the use of drawings from
Anatomy of the Human Body, by Henry Gray, 28th Edition, 1966.

Miss Craig's Jacket: Saks Fifth Avenue, New York
Clothes Stylist: Freddy Plimpton
Hair Stylist: Michael Fitzpatrick
Photographer: Steve Manville
Designer: R. Scudellari
Created under the personal editorship of Phyllis Cerf

Copyright © 1970 by Marjorie Craig
All rights reserved under International and Pan-American Copyright Conventions.
Published in the United States by Random House, Inc., New York, and simultaneously
in Canada by Random House of Canada Limited, Toronto.
Library of Congress Catalog Card Number: 73-102904
Manufactured in the United States of America

Contents

Introduction

We have too long been just plain ignorant about facial muscles. This lack of knowledge has caused us to accept as fact all sorts of mumbo jumbo about our faces. It has been said, for instance, that (1) one must never move the muscles of the face, for it is movement that causes wrinkles; (2) what we are and what we feel eventually show up as lines on our faces and there's nothing we can do about it — it's fate; (3) massaging, rubbing, and/or patting the face will iron out wrinkles — and keep them ironed out. None of these statements would seem to be true in light of what research has shown me about the structure of the face.

Under the skin of the human face — be it male or female — there are bones, blood vessels, connective tissue, fat, nerves and muscles. It is the bones of the skull, and the muscles which cover it, that give the face its contour. It is the tonus condition of these facial muscles which determines whether or not the skin of the face is flabby or firm in appearance.

Muscles of the face, as well as muscles of the body, are made up of bundles of cylindrical fibers. A single muscle may contain as few as three, or as many as 165 fibers — each fiber working independently in the sense that only when one fiber is fully contracted (shortened) is the next fiber triggered to work. To tone a muscle completely, *all* of its fibers must be used. When you move a muscle quickly, gravity and/or momentum often does part of the moving job for you. This means that you do not need — and therefore do not use — the total number of fibers available, so a portion of the muscle remains unused. The individual fibers of a muscle cannot be partially contracted — they are either contracted fully or not at all.

Each muscle of the face and the body is there to do a job. We have, for instance, a muscle that opens the eye, and one that closes the eye; a muscle to lift the eyebrows, one to lower the eyebrows. In other words, nature has provided a muscle to do a specific job, and another to do the exact opposite. The muscles that do opposite jobs from one another are called "antagonistic muscles," but in actuality they are not antagonistic to one another — they work as a team. When one contracts (shortens) to do a "moving" job, the other relaxes (lengthens) to the same extent its teammate has contracted, thus allowing smooth movements. If one muscle is constantly contracted, it follows that its antagonistic muscle must be constantly relaxed. This constant state of either contraction or relaxation may produce an expression on your face you love, but it is this "set expression" that causes a pair of muscles to lose tone, for neither one is being used to its fullest extent. The only way to keep a muscle healthy and in tone is to use it to its fullest capacity. Sagging skin and/or deep furrows are indications that facial muscles are out of condition — that is, they have lost their tonus. What, exactly, is tonus? Tonus is a normal state of slight but continuous contraction in a muscle.

A muscle with tonus is said to have elasticity. What is elasticity? It is the property which enables muscles to regain their original size and shape after having been stretched. The skin also has an elastic quality, and it is the condition of the muscles beneath it that helps determine the tonus condition of the skin. A firm face is a symbol of youth, but a firm face need not be the property solely of the young. If muscles of the body can be brought back to tone — and they can be — so can muscles of the face, and by the same means: exercise.

The thirty exercises that make up my face-saving program are based on using muscles the way nature intended they be used in order to counterbalance the aging effects of gravity — which is constantly pulling facial muscles downward — and also to counterbalance "set expression" patterns which weaken facial muscles. The expression muscles of the face, of which there are twenty-six, are known anatomically as voluntary muscles — voluntary muscles being those under the control of one's will.

Every muscle has a beginning and an end. Its beginning and its end are attached to something. In the body each end of the muscle is generally attached to bone; this is not true, however, of muscles of the face. Their connections are many and varied. For instance, the muscle which produces a frown is attached to bone. As that muscle narrows, some of its fibers terminate by attaching themselves to the eye-closing muscle, while its other fibers terminate in the skin of the forehead. Thus we see that the muscles of the face attach to bone, attach to other muscles, and also attach to skin. Because muscles of the face are attached to skin, it is their function to move skin. *So don't be afraid to move facial muscles.* Out-of-tone muscles first bring a sagging and crepy texture to the skin which eventually forms into lines and wrinkles. Lines and wrinkles can also be brought to the superficial skin of the face by illness, deep emotional stress, the sun. I advise my clients not to lie in the sun without either first covering their faces with an emollient that filters out the harmful rays of the sun or using a sun hat or umbrella. In my opinion, there is really nothing that dries and ages the skin as quickly as overexposing the skin to the sun.

If you've begun to notice a little sagging skin, a telltale line here and there, as you look at your face in the mirror, there's one thing you can be sure of — it's not going to get any better, unless you do something about it. Whether your problems started with the sun, with gravity's downward pull on your facial muscles and skin, or with a habit of fixing your face into a set expression, my facial exercises can be of help to you, as they have been to my pupils. In every instance, regardless of age, they feel they have gotten results. Some of my pupils said their skin was better almost at once — that is, in a matter of days. I personally saw small improvements in my pupils' faces in a couple of weeks. The improvement became quite apparent to everyone — to me, to them, to friends, to husbands, to wives — during a four- or five-month period — and it's still going on. This is not to say that my pupils look as if they had had their faces lifted, but as one commented, they no longer look as if they needed to have it done, either.

Certain of my pupils are still too young to have developed wrinkles on their faces, but they are now doing the exercises as a preventive measure, and even they have found an immediate benefit: without exception, all of their complexions have shown improvement. Incidentally, when you first start doing the facial exercises, even if you are past a "certain" age, don't be surprised if an occasional blemish appears. You'll be bringing natural oils to the tissues which may not have had them for years. This "adolescent" disorder disappears after the first week or so, once the tissues and the natural oils have become reacquainted.

Once you've learned the exercises, you can do them all in about fifteen minutes a day. They need not be done at one sitting, nor is there any magic in performing them in a particular order. The only important thing is to do them until you see the results *you* want.

I have presented, along with each exercise, the anatomical explanation, location and function of each of the twenty-six voluntary facial muscles you will be using. My purpose for doing this is to enable you to learn *what* muscles you are moving, and to assure you that you are moving them "naturally." With this knowledge, you will discover that *you* are the magician that can bring about changes in your face — and just doing what comes naturally is a way to grow older with grace and dignity.

Before You Begin...

1. All these exercises should be done with a mirror in hand, or while sitting or standing in front of a mirror. In time, it will be possible for you to do these exercises correctly without a mirror, but in the beginning you will need to check muscle movements of the face.

2. These exercises can also be done while lying on a slant board (see photo below), to bring even better circulation to the face.

3. Concentrate on keeping muscles not being exercised as relaxed as possible.

4. All exercises should be done slowly and deliberately, with the exerciser being consciously aware of every movement that is made.

5. If you feel you do not need to do all the facial exercises, you may choose not to use the six-day learning plan. If this is the case, turn directly to the exercises for the area you are most concerned about. Then check the "What's Your Problem?" chart to see if there are other exercises you should be doing to solve your facial problems.

6. Medical men who have examined my exercises prior to publication feel that a manual such as this, with description of the mechanics of performance of exercises of the muscles of the face, could be made useful to people who wished to have written directions to follow to improve facial muscle functions before or after surgery; after injuries, or a spontaneous loss, such as Bell's palsy. Persons who have had, or are about to have any facial surgery, or the like, should show the exercises to their personal physician before beginning the program. Get his advice as to your individual ability to move through the program.

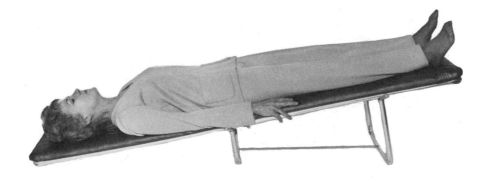

Chart: What's Your Problem?

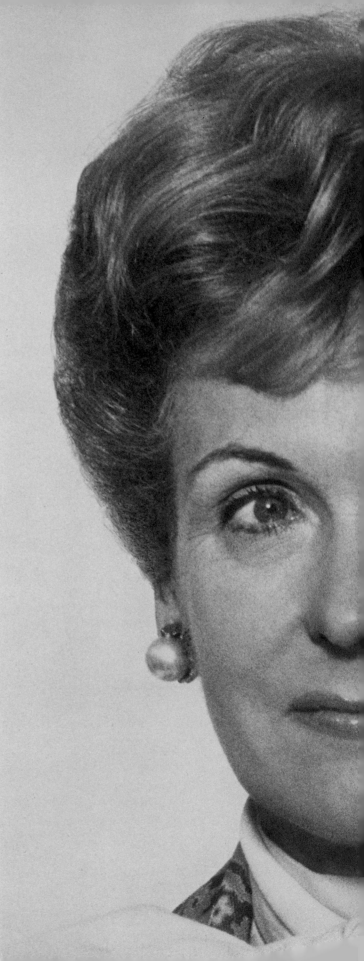

Forehead/Scalp

Lines across forehead?
See: Corrugator, Frontalis, Occipitalis, Procerus

Frown lines between brows?
See: Corrugator, Frontalis

Sag between brows?
See: Frontalis, Procerus

Eyelids

Crepy, droopy, puffy upper eyelids?
See: Corrugator, Frontalis, Levator palpebrae, Orbicularis oculi, Tensor tarsi

Crow's-feet?
See: Caput zygomaticum, Frontalis, Masseter, Orbicularis oculi, Temporalis, Zygomaticus

Hollow circles under eyes?
See: Caput angulare, Caput infra-orbitale, Caput zygomaticum, Orbicularis oculi, Tensor tarsi

Puffiness under eyes?
See: Caninus, Caput angulare, Caput infra-orbitale, Caput zygomaticum, Orbicularis oculi, Tensor tarsi, Zygomaticus

Squint lines under eyes?
See: Caninus, Caput angulare, Caput infra-orbitale, Caput zygomaticum, Orbicularis oculi, Zygomaticus

Nose

Lines and wrinkles at bridge of nose?
See: Caput angulare, Corrugator, Frontalis, Orbicularis oculi, Procerus

Sunburst of wrinkles between bridge of nose and nostrils?
See: Caput angulare, Frontalis

Deep grooves at nose wings?
See: Caninus, Caput angulare

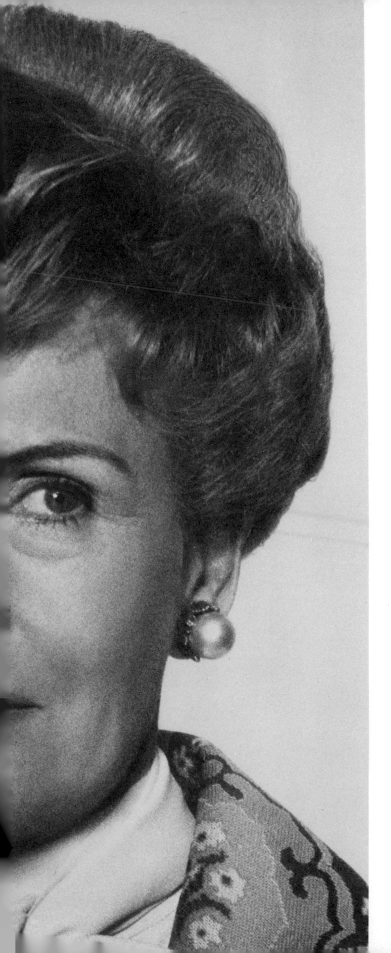

Cheeks

Droopy, sunken and/or wrinkled cheeks?
See: Buccinator, Caninus, Caput angulare, Caput infra-orbitale, Caput zygomaticum, Risorius, Zygomaticus

Furrows from nose to mouth?
See: Caninus, Zygomaticus

Wrinkles in front of ears?
See: Digastricus, Masseter, Pterygoids, Temporalis

Furrows from cheekbone to lower jawbone?
See: Digastricus, Masseter, Pterygoids, Temporalis

Dimpled hollows in cheekbone area?
See: Buccinator, Caput zygomaticum, Zygomaticus

Upper Lip & Mouth

Vertical lines on upper lip?
See: Buccinator, Caninus, Caput angulare, Caput infra-orbitale, Caput zygomaticum, Orbicularis oris, Risorius, Zygomaticus

Pouches at corners of upper lip?
See: Buccinator, Caninus, Orbicularis oris, Risorius, Triangularis, Zygomaticus

Smile lines at sides of mouth?
See: Orbicularis oris, Platysma, Quadratus labii inferioris, Risorius, Triangularis

Chin & Jawline

Crepy chin?
See: Buccinator, Mentalis, Orbicularis oris, Platysma, Quadratus labii inferioris, Risorius, Triangularis

Hollowed area beneath lower lip?
See: Caninus, Platysma, Quadratus labii inferioris, Risorius, Triangularis

Jowls?
See: Digastricus, Masseter, Mylohyoideus, Platysma, Pterygoids, Temporalis

Furrows from mouth corners to jawline?
See: Buccinator, Mentalis, Quadratus labii inferioris, Triangularis

Under-Chin & Throat

Double chin?
See: All neck muscles, Digastricus, Masseter, Mentalis, Mylohyoideus, Platysma, Pterygoids, Sternocleidomastoideus, Temporalis, Triangularis .

Crepy neck?
See: All neck muscles, Platysma, Sternocleidomastoideus, Triangularis

Thick neck?
See: All neck muscles, Platysma, Sternocleidomastoideus, Triangularis

The 6-Day Face-Saving Program

The Face-Saving Program consists of 30 comprehensive exercises grouped for easy learning and convenient reference by facial areas,* starting with the forehead and scalp and systematically working downward through the face, muscle by muscle, to the under-chin and throat.

The learning program is arranged so that all facial exercises are introduced in six days (a facial area a day), and once an exercise is introduced, it becomes part of all subsequent days' programs.

Each exercise has been given a number and a name. A chart listing exercise numbers and names along with the suggested number of repetitions is provided at the beginning of each section to guide you through the program day by day. The exercise name is intended to serve you as a memory aid so that eventually, by using the 6th Day chart as a check list, you can do the exercises without reading through the book page by page.

If your muscles are not tired after doing an exercise for the given number of times, there is no reason for not doing more, if you so desire. You might get quicker results if you do—and you will not develop muscle soreness. Soreness is brought about by muscle strain. My exercises are based on moving the muscles the way nature intended, and therefore do not cause strain.

Muscles are moved by "telegraphing" move messages via nerves to the brain. If you encounter difficulty in getting certain muscles to move on demand, be assured you are not unique — and something can be done about it. The quickest and easiest way to get a muscle moving is to use it in conjunction with a familiar facial expression. Once the muscle has been moved, the "message" channel is open and you can instantly use it again for an exercise. With this "telegraph" system in mind, I have given "the use (of each muscle) in expressive action" on the page opposite each exercise. By all means, use this "expressive" method until you've gained total control over your muscles and can make them move by willing them to do so.

By experimenting and testing, I discovered that results came more quickly to those who did the exercises very slowly. Upon thinking about it, the reason for this became apparent. To move a muscle slowly requires more control than to move it quickly. With more control, more fibers of a muscle come into use. The more fibers that are used, the more thoroughly a muscle is exercised. The more thoroughly a muscle is exercised, the more quickly a muscle is toned. Remember that — go to work — and you'll soon be looking at a younger-looking you.

*(1) Forehead and Scalp (2) The Eyelid (3) Nose and Cheek (4) Lower Cheek and Lips (5) Chin and Jawline (6) Under-Chin and Throat

1st Day
Forehead & Scalp

Drooping eyebrows and puffy skin above the eyes
are good indicators that you really do need
to do the exercises in this section—even
if you have a smooth forehead.

People with deep forehead wrinkles will also
benefit from these exercises—but you
knew that, didn't you?

Once you've learned the exercises, you can
do them any time, anywhere that's convenient.
When you begin to see the results you want,
there will be no need for you to do them
every day, but in the beginning you should,
so that you'll see improvement and
will want to keep them up.

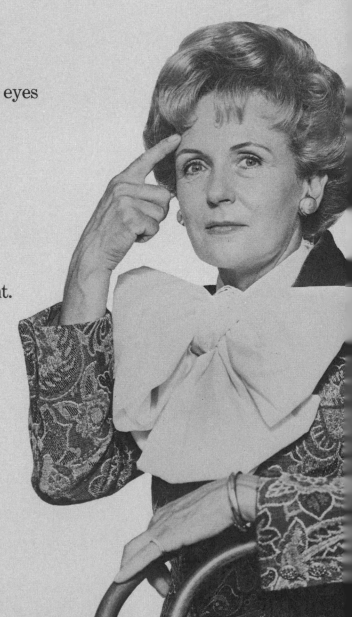

14

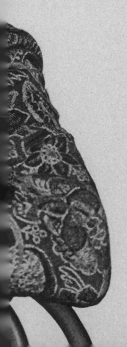

The 1st Day's Program

Pages 16-21

Do:

Exercise 1	*The Scalp Raiser*	*20 times*
Exercise 2	*The Defrowner*	*5 times*
Exercise 3	*The Bridge Crosser*	*5 times*

The muscles involved are: Frontalis, Occipitalis, Corrugator supercilii, Procerus.

1 The Scalp Raiser

TO SMOOTH THE BROW

The Muscle:

The *Frontalis* (fron tā' lis) raises the eyebrows, maintains the smoothness of the skin between the eyebrows, and additionally, pulls the scalp forward. Its fibers extend upward from eyebrow to hairline, joining with the tendinous fibers of the scalp. When the Frontalis is contracted to do its eyebrow-raising job, its fibers shorten, and in so doing, momentarily wrinkle the skin across the forehead. Removing these wrinkles is the function of the *Occipitalis* (ok sip i tā'lis) muscle, which is located at the other end of those tendinous fibers of the scalp.

As the Frontalis relaxes (lengthens), the Occipitalis contracts (shortens), and thus returns the scalp to its normal resting position. When both of these muscles are "in good working order," deeply engraved transverse wrinkles will fade from the brow. To get these two muscles moving smoothly in conjunction with each other, you may need the help of gravity. (See opposite page.)

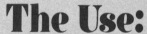

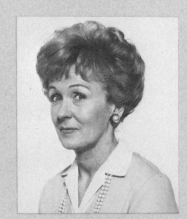

The Use:

IN EXPRESSIVE ACTION: The Frontalis produces an expression we associate with being surprised. Raise your eyebrows. Look in the mirror. Don't be surprised that it makes it easier to do these exercises by first assuming the appropriate facial expression.

16

The Exercise:

Holding a hand mirror during this exercise will help you to see—and thus isolate—the movements of the forehead and scalp muscles.

1. Lie down on a bed. To get gravity's help, lie with head hanging over the edge of bed.

2. Raise your eyebrows as high as you can.

3. Return the eyebrows to normal position.

DO EXERCISE **20** TIMES, COUNTING EACH TIME YOU RAISE YOUR BROWS.

2 The Defrowner
TO HELP ALLEVIATE VERTICAL FROWN LINES

The Muscle:
The *Corrugator supercilii* (kor'u gā tor su per sil' i ī) pulls the eyebrows toward one another and downward to the eyes. In so doing, it brings vertical lines to the skin between the brows and produces the "frown" expression associated with suffering and perplexity. The two Corrugators are placed at the medial ends of the eyebrows. Some of their fibers intermingle with muscles surrounding the eyes and others attach to the skin of the forehead.

Frown lines deepen and become a permanent part of facial expression when the Frontalis and Corrugator muscles are not equally toned to interact with each other as nature intended they should. When properly toned, the Frontalis automatically returns the eyebrows to their natural spread-apart position as the Corrugator is relaxed from its "frowning" contraction.

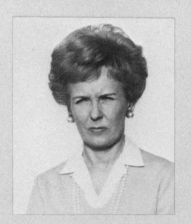

The Use:
IN EXPRESSIVE ACTION:
Look perplexed. Peer off into the distance as if to see something that's hard for you to see. Look in the mirror. Have your eyebrows gone down? If they have, you've used the Corrugator.

The Exercise:

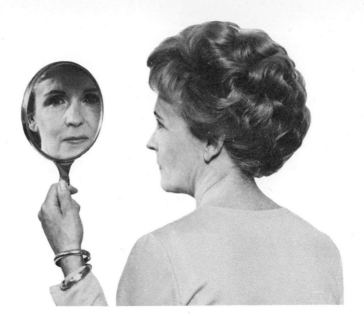

1. Face mirror squarely,
   with eyes open.

2. Pull your eyebrows way down over your eyes.
   In other words, really frown.

3. Frown so hard that it will feel as though you were
   trying to get your eyebrows
   to meet one another.
   Think "frown" as you frown.

4. Then lift your eyebrows as high —
   and open your eyes as wide — as you can.

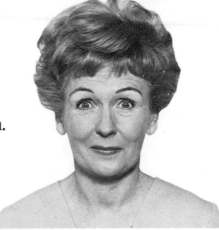

DO EXERCISE **5**
TIMES, COUNTING EACH TIME YOU FROWN.

19

3 The Bridge Crosser

TO HELP ALLEVIATE TRANSVERSE LINES ON THE BRIDGE OF THE NOSE

The Muscle:

The *Procerus* (pro sē' rus) draws the skin of the central part of the forehead downward, along with the medial ends of the eyebrows. This pyramidal muscle of the nose begins at the lower part of the nasal bone and extends upward to terminate between the brows. At the brow its fibers intermingle with the blended fibers of the right and left Frontales. Wrinkles are brought to the bridge of the nose by the Procerus. The blended fibers of the Frontalis remove them. Paradoxically, you will have to consciously bring wrinkles to the bridge of the nose in order to activate—and thus tone—the central fibers of the Frontalis.

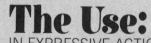

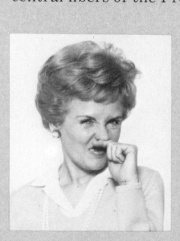

The Use:

IN EXPRESSIVE ACTION:
In order to more easily isolate the movement of the Procerus, wrinkle up your nose as if you were about to sneeze —or were indicating something smelled bad.

The Exercise:

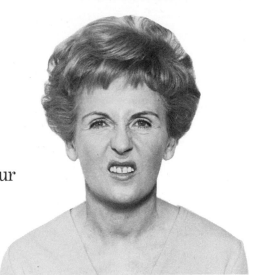

1. Relax the forehead. Wrinkle nose up until the lines across the bridge of your nose are deep, or at least apparent.

2. Now, try to make the lines deeper by drawing the ends of your eyebrows 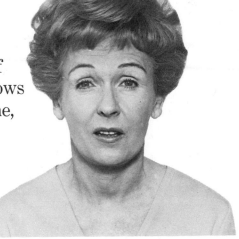 down toward the bridge of your nose.

3. Remove the creases from the bridge of your nose by slowly lifting your eyebrows as high as you can, and at the same time, release the wrinkles from your nose.

DO EXERCISE **5** TIMES, COUNTING EACH TIME YOU BRING CREASES TO NOSE.

2nd Day
The Eyelid

People worry about doing eyelid exercises. They reason that moving eyelid skin as they squinted and laughed was the beginning of their eyelid problems — and naturally wonder how further moving of eyelid muscles is going to take their eyelid problems away. The answer is simple: All the eyelid muscles can be kept in tone only by using them ALL. Most of us stop using ALL of the fibers in eyelid muscles when we stop making childhood faces.

Actually, the eye-area muscles are very small and will respond to exercise rather quickly. Some fibers of the eyelid muscles are embedded in the skin, so it follows that as the muscles are toned, the skin will tone also.

When you have learned the eyelid exercises, you can do them anywhere, any time, as often as you like. I have found that doing the eye squeezes in bed is very relaxing to the eyes.

An additional hint: While walking around all day, remember to use your eye-opening muscle again and again and again. You'll be glad you did.

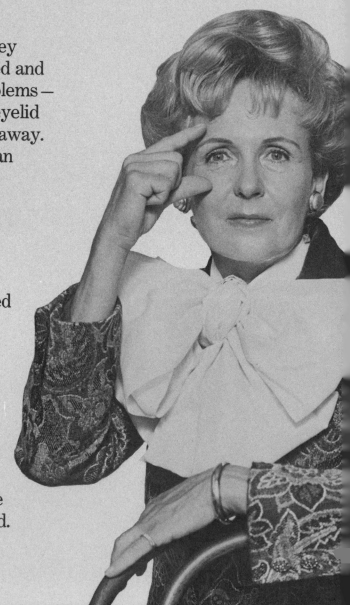

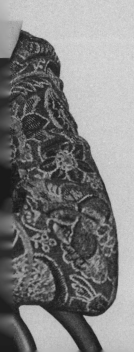

The 2nd Day's Program

Pages 24-35

Do:

Exercise 1	The Scalp Raiser	*20 times*
Exercise 2	The Defrowner	*5 times*
Exercise 3	The Bridge Crosser	*5 times*

New Exercises:

Exercise 4	The Eye Squeeze	*5 times*
Exercise 5	The Cryer	*3 times*
Exercise 6	The Eye Stretcher	*3 times*
Exercise 7	The Bag Trick	*3 times*
Exercise 8	The Eye Opener	*3 times*
Exercise 9	The Eye Resister	*5 times*

Muscles involved: Orbicularis oculi, Tensor tarsi, Levator palpebrae superioris.

4 The Eye Squeeze
TO HELP TONE UPPER AND LOWER EYELIDS

The Muscle:
The *Orbicularis oculi* (or bik ū lā′ ris   ok′ ū lī) helps bring the eyebrows down toward the eyes, but its primary function is to close the eyelids. It will close them gently—for sleep, emphatically—for a wink, or strongly—to squeeze out all light. The *orbital* portion (one of three in this sphincter muscle) encircles the eye socket without interruption, with some of its fibers spreading to the forehead, temple, cheek and eyebrow. The only time you use all the spreading fibers of the Orbicularis oculi is when you squeeze your eyes tightly shut. This causes (though you can't see it) skin to be drawn toward the eyes from the forehead, temple and cheek. Is that good? It is if you want to get rid of upper and lower eyelid droop caused by out-of-tone muscle.

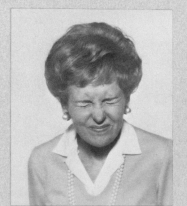

The Use:
IN EXPRESSIVE ACTION: Close your eyes. Close them tight. No peeking until I say "Ready"—and you will have surely used the orbital fibers of your Orbicularis oculi. Ready!

24

The Exercise:

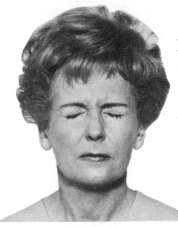
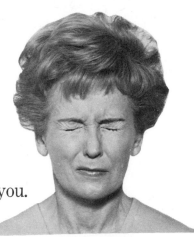

1. Close your eyes into a tight squeeze.

2. Then think of squeezing your eyes even more tightly closed — and do it. Let your cheek muscles help you.

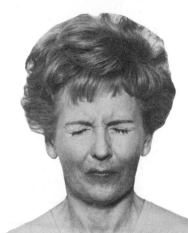
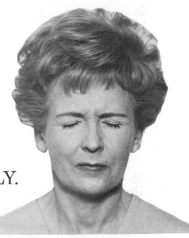

3. Now, think of releasing the squeeze — and do it.

DO IT SLOWLY.

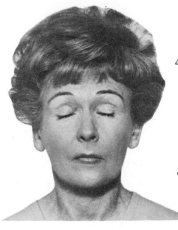
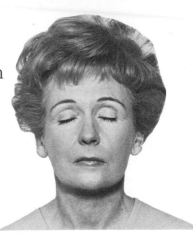

4. Lift the eyebrows and stretch the upper lids as wide as you can over your closed eyes. Really stretch those eyelids.

5. Slowly release the stretch.

DO EXERCISE **5** TIMES, COUNTING EACH TIME YOU SQUEEZE EYES CLOSED.

5 The Cryer

TO HELP ALLEVIATE DROOPING UPPER EYELIDS

The Muscle:
The second portion of the Orbicularis oculi is known as the *Tensor tarsi* (ten' sor tar' sī). Its function is to help keep the eyelid in contact with the eyeball. It also draws the tear-receiving canals to a favorable position to receive tears, and helps to pump the tears into the nasal passage.

The Tensor tarsi is not a voluntary muscle—that is to say, it is not activated by will power, but by body needs. So... unless you cry a lot, it will be good to put your eyes in the crying position, and thus help to smooth out the little puffs at the inside corners of the eyelids.

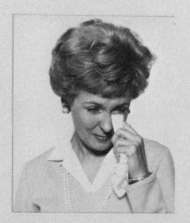

The Use:
IN EXPRESSIVE ACTION: They say, "Crying is for babies, not for grownups," so squeeze your eyes as if you were crying. Then someone might say, "You have pretty eyes, baby!"

26

The Exercise:

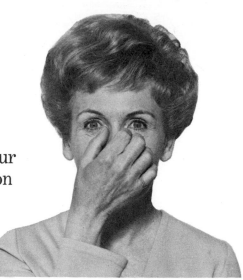

1. Look in the mirror and place your thumb and index finger lightly on the inside corners of your eyes.

2. Close your eyes. Keeping cheek muscles relaxed, squeeze the corners of your eyelids in toward fingers. When you've squeezed in as far as you think the muscle will go...

Squeeze harder.

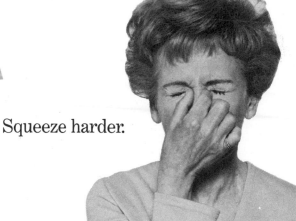

3. Slowly release the squeeze You may feel a little teary. If you do, you can be sure you've done the exercise correctly.

DO EXERCISE **3** TIMES, COUNTING EACH TIME YOU SQUEEZE.

6 The Eye Stretcher
TO HELP TONE UPPER EYELIDS

The Muscle: The third
portion of the *Orbicularis oculi* is the
palpebral — known to us as our upper
and lower eyelids. We tend to permit
gravity to close our eyes rather than
to activate the eyelid-closing muscles
to do the job. This causes eyelids to
become crepy. The following exercise
will help to tone the upper eyelids and
the drooping upper brow — and in addition,
the stretching will make your eyes feel good.

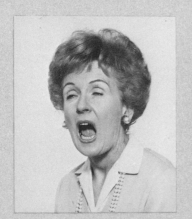

The Use:
IN EXPRESSIVE ACTION:
"Excuse my yawn, but with a
yawn I not only stretch my
mouth, I also stretch my eyelids
...and that's how I 'naturally'
use the muscle you'll now be
exercising."

28

The Exercise:

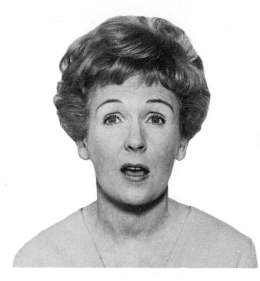

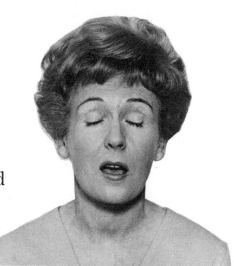

1. Open your mouth slightly. Raise your eyebrows and close your eyes.

2. As you raise the eyebrows up, stretch downward with your eyelids. Feel as if you're trying to get the greatest possible distance between your eyebrows and lashes. Hold the stretch for the count of 10.

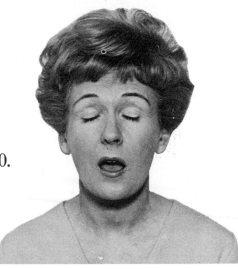

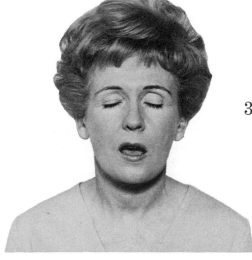

3. Very slowly and consciously, release the pressure on your eyelids and relax the lids, returning eyebrows to normal position.

DO EXERCISE **3** TIMES, COUNTING EACH TIME UPPER LID IS RELAXED.

7 The Bag Trick

TO TONE UNDER-EYE AREA

The Muscle:

The *palpebral* portion of the *Orbicularis oculi* of the lower lid is rarely called upon to function—i.e., help close the eyes. As babies we used both our upper and lower lids to close our eyes—and if you'd like that "baby" look again, you'd better start using your lower lids.

First do the exercise with your eyes closed, as described on the opposite page. As your lower eyelids get stronger, open your eyes and see if you can bring your lower lids up with your eyes wide open. Then you'll know you're exercising your lower lid eye-closing muscle as it should be exercised.

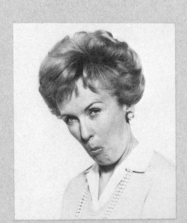

The Use:

IN EXPRESSIVE ACTION:
If you thought someone was trying to fool you, you might pull your jaw down without opening your lips and squint at them to let them know you weren't fooled. If you squinted this way, you'd definitely have to use the palpebral portion of your lower lid—I'm not fooling; don't look at me that way.

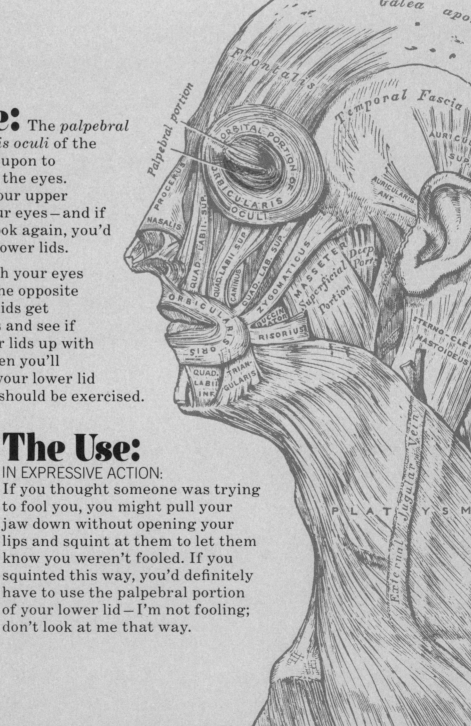

30

The Exercise:

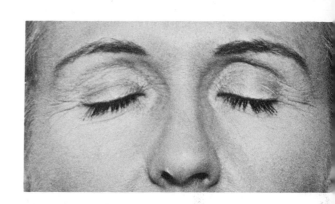

1. Close your eyes gently, as you do when closing them for sleep.

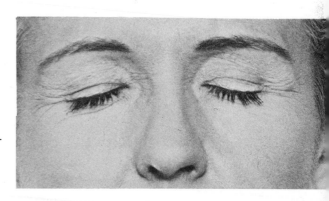

2. Keep your upper lids closed and as relaxed as possible. Now, think about lifting the lower lids upward—and do it—keeping all other facial muscles as relaxed as possible.

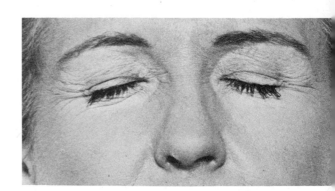

3. Hold the lower lids in this contracted, stretched position for the count of 5. Then slowly release the contraction, allowing lower lids to return to a relaxed position for the count of 5.

DO EXERCISE **3**
TIMES, COUNTING EACH TIME YOU LIFT LOWER LIDS.

31

8 The Eye Opener
TO HELP ALLEVIATE DROOPING UPPER LIDS

The Muscle: The *Levator palpebrae superioris* (lē vā′ tor pal′ pē brē su pē ri ō′ ris) is generally anatomically classed with the muscles of the eye, and I suppose literally it is a muscle that helps us to see, for its function is to raise the upper eyelids to their "open" position and to keep them raised despite gravity's downward pull. The Levator palpebrae superioris terminates in the deep surface of the skin of the upper eyelid. Though the action part of this muscle is behind the eyes, its function finally determines the tonus condition of your upper eyelid.

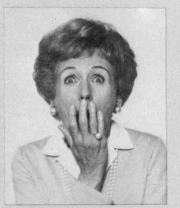

The Use:
IN EXPRESSIVE ACTION:
If you can't believe what your eyes see, you're apt to open them wide. But to open them still wider, stare at yourself in front of a mirror until you see the white of your eye above the iris.

32

The Exercise:

1. Stand close to a mirror and raise your eyebrows as high as you can, and keep them raised.

2. Keeping eyebrows raised, lower your upper lids about halfway, to cover a portion of the iris.

3. Now, think about your eye-opening muscle, and activate it to open your upper lids again. Open them all the way to show white above the iris.

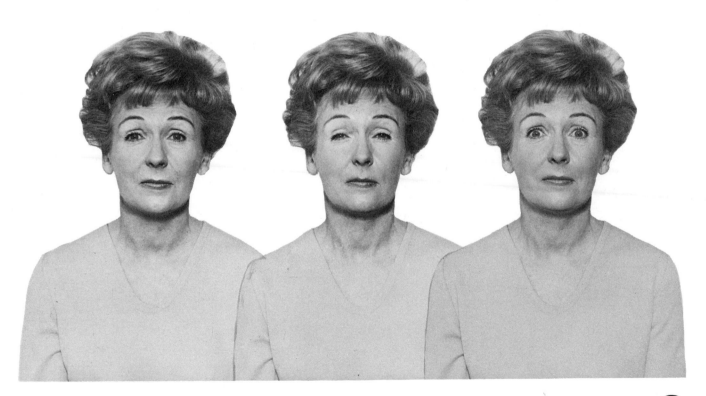

DO EXERCISE **3** TIMES, COUNTING EACH TIME YOU LIFT UPPER LIDS.

9 The Eye Resister

TO SMOOTH OUT THE "CROW'S-FEET" AREA OF THE EYES

The Muscle:

The *Orbicularis oculi* is the eye-closing muscle. The *Levator palpebrae superioris* is the eye-opening muscle. In anatomical language it is said that these two muscles work in opposition to each other. This means that as the Orbicularis oculi contracts (shortens), the Levator palpebrae superioris relaxes (lengthens) to the same degree, and vice versa. To bring these "opposing" muscles into tone more quickly, you need to consciously control the eye-closing and eye-opening movements and thus make sure the muscles—not gravity— are taking care of your "eye" job.

All the eye exercises will help to improve the looks of the crow's-feet area, but this special little exercise, once you've gotten the feel of it, is one you can do almost anywhere, any time—and you should.

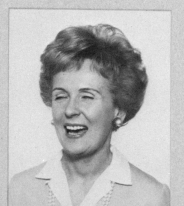

The Use:

IN EXPRESSIVE ACTION: If you ever pretended your eyes were closed, but in truth you were peering through your eyelashes to see what was going on, you were simultaneously using your eye-opening and eye-closing muscles. Do it again!

34

The Exercise:

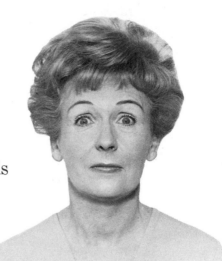

1. Stand close to a mirror. Raise your eyebrows and lift upper lids until you see the whites of your eyes above the iris.

2. Slowly begin to bring your upper and lower lids together until you appear slit-eyed. Think about both lids resisting each other as you bring them together.

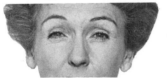

To do this properly, you will need to concentrate. The upper lids should not move down at a faster rate than the lower lids move up.

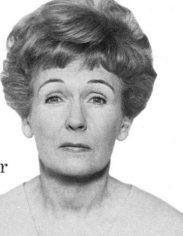

3. Now, slowly open your eyes, again thinking of resisting as you concentrate on moving the upper and lower lids apart at the same slow pace.

DO EXERCISE **5**
TIMES, COUNTING EACH TIME LIDS ARE BROUGHT TOGETHER.

3rd Day
Nose & Cheek

The contour of the cheek is affected by the way you move your mouth—for curious as it may seem, your mouth-moving muscles help give your upper cheek its form. To the eye your cheeks may look firm, but unless they feel firm to the touch, it's a cinch they lack tone. Other tell-tale signs of poor tone are: deep hollows under the eyes, deep grooves between nostrils and lip corners, and crinkling of skin around the upper and lower lip.

Why exercise the nose? Some doctors say the nose grows longer as we grow older. It's highly possible, for gravity does pull everything downward—and why should the nose be an exception! Exercise will keep the nose from becoming pinched-looking.

Do the nose and cheek exercises regularly every day for the rest of your life. These muscles contribute greatly to the tonus condition of your whole face.

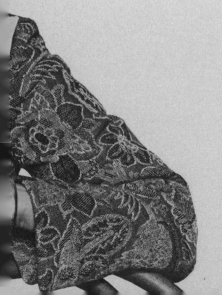

The 3rd Day's Program

Pages 38-49

Do:

Exercise 1	The Scalp Raiser	*20 times*
Exercise 2	The Defrowner	*5 times*
Exercise 3	The Bridge Crosser	*5 times*
Exercise 4	The Eye Squeeze	*5 times*
Exercise 5	The Cryer	*3 times*
Exercise 6	The Eye Stretcher	*3 times*
Exercise 7	The Bag Trick	*3 times*
Exercise 8	The Eye Opener	*3 times*
Exercise 9	The Eye Resister	*5 times*

New Exercises:

Exercise 10	The Nose Wrinkler	*5 times*
Exercise 11	The Cheek Raiser	*5 times*
Exercise 12	The Lid Lifter	*5 times*
Exercise 13	The Big Laugh	*5 times*
Exercise 14	Raising a Furrow	*2 times*
Exercise 15	The Teeth Clencher	*10 times*

Muscles involved: Caput angulare, Caput infra-orbitale, Caput zygomaticum of the Quadratus labii superioris, Zygomaticus, Caninus, Masseter.

10 The Nose Wrinkler
TO FILL IN HOLLOWS BETWEEN NOSE AND CHEEKS

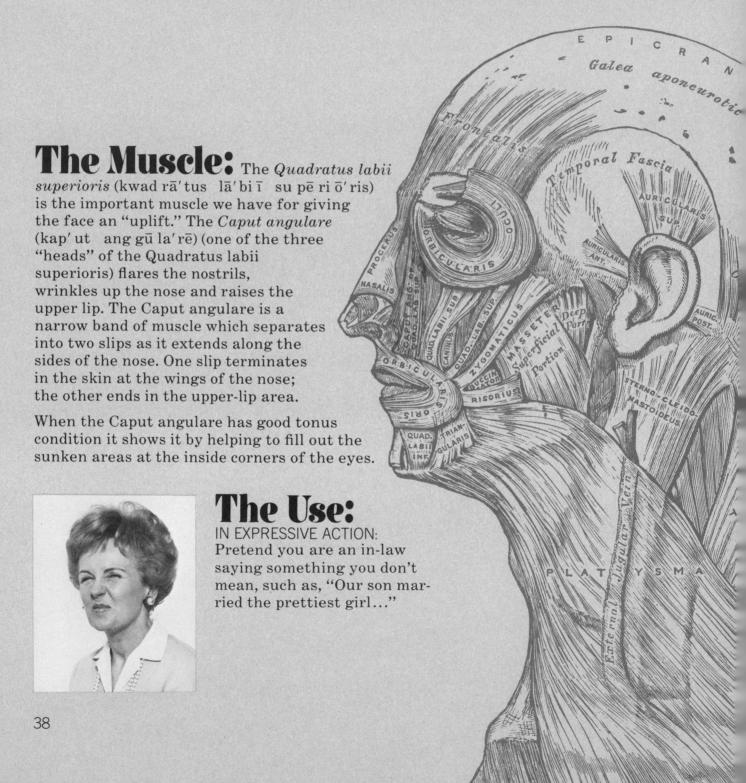

The Muscle:
The *Quadratus labii superioris* (kwad rā′tus lā′bi ī su pē ri ō′ris) is the important muscle we have for giving the face an "uplift." The *Caput angulare* (kap′ut ang gū la′rē) (one of the three "heads" of the Quadratus labii superioris) flares the nostrils, wrinkles up the nose and raises the upper lip. The Caput angulare is a narrow band of muscle which separates into two slips as it extends along the sides of the nose. One slip terminates in the skin at the wings of the nose; the other ends in the upper-lip area.

When the Caput angulare has good tonus condition it shows it by helping to fill out the sunken areas at the inside corners of the eyes.

The Use:
IN EXPRESSIVE ACTION: Pretend you are an in-law saying something you don't mean, such as, "Our son married the prettiest girl..."

The Exercise:

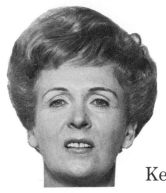

1. Look directly into a mirror. Open mouth slightly. Flare the nostrils of your nose.

Keeping nostrils flared...

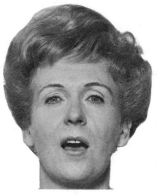

2. Slowly wrinkle your nose. Wrinkle it up as far as it will go. (If you do it correctly, your nasal passages will feel opened, and your relaxed upper lip will have been drawn upward.) Now...

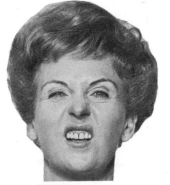

3. Concentrate on that pulled-up upper lip...

4. And use it to pull down...

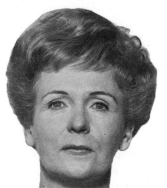

5. Pull your upper lip down slowly until your nose is unwrinkled and back to its normal position.

DO EXERCISE **5** TIMES, COUNTING EACH TIME YOU WRINKLE NOSE UP.

11 The Cheek Raiser
TO LIFT AND FIRM THE UPPER-CHEEK AREA

The Muscle: The *Caput infra-orbitale* (kap′ut in′fra or bi tā′lē) lifts the cheeks in order to raise the upper lip. This middle head of the Quadratus labii superioris originates at the cheekbone below the center of the eye socket; its fibers travel downward to terminate in the upper lip. Its fibers assist in forming the furrow that passes from the side of the nose to the upper lip. The more toned this muscle, the more lifted the cheeks. Muscles that are lifted don't sag to make deep furrows.

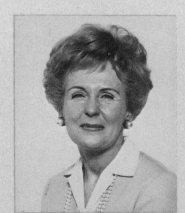

The Use:

IN EXPRESSIVE ACTION: This is the muscle you would use to produce a sincerely insincere saccharine smile as a companion for little white lies such as, "But, darling, I *love* fake diamonds."

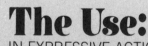

The Exercise:

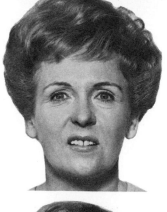

1. Look directly into a mirror. Flare the nostrils of your nose. Keep them flared.

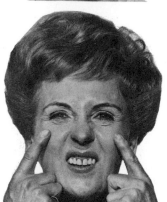

2. Now, raise the "apple-cheek" area of your cheeks up toward your eyes. Put your index fingers on this raised "apple-cheek" area.

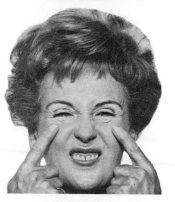

3. Tighten the cheek muscles under your fingers. Keep tightening this part of your cheeks until your upper lip curls up to the point where it almost touches your nose.

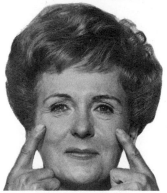

4. Slowly return curled lip to normal position.

DO EXERCISE **5** TIMES, COUNTING EACH TIME YOU CURL UP YOUR UPPER LIP.

41

1² The Lid Lifter

TO FILL IN HOLLOWS IN CHEEKBONE AREA

The Muscle:

The *Caput zygomaticum* (kap′ut   zī gō mat′i kum) pulls up the corner of the lips, and when it does, the whole cheek goes up with it. This third head of the Quadratus labii superioris originates at the cheekbone at the outer corner of the eye, where its fibers intermingle with the eye-closing muscle. From its origin, it follows an oblique path down the cheek and terminates in the skin of the upper lip.

The three heads of the Quadratus labii superioris act together, as well as separately. When all three are in tone, the upper cheek will stay up instead of sagging, and thereby lessen the depth of the furrow between the nose and the corner of the lip.

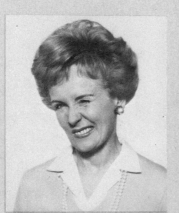

The Use:

IN EXPRESSIVE ACTION: If it's really activated, the Caput zygomaticum can help push the lower eyelid closed in the wink of an eye. Want to prove it? Wink!

42

The Exercise:

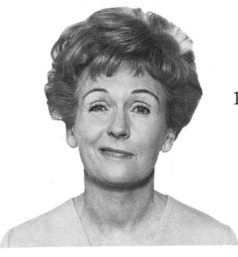

1. Get close to a mirror. Raise your eyebrows. Make a crooked grin with the right side of your mouth. Hold that position throughout exercise.

2. Place right index finger on cheek below outer corner of right eye. Your finger is now resting on the muscle to be exercised.

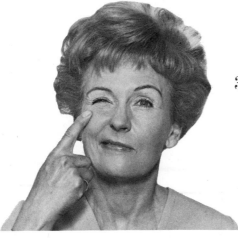

3. Think about this muscle and use it to slowly push the lower lid of your right eye closed. Hold. Then slowly return to normal position.

4. Repeat all the above movements with left eye.

DO EXERCISE **5** TIMES, COUNTING EACH TIME YOU CLOSE RIGHT EYE.

13 The Big Laugh

TO LIFT THE CHEEKS AND THE CORNERS OF THE MOUTH

The Muscle:

The *Zygomaticus* (zī gō mat′ i kus) is the muscle that draws up the corners of your mouth so you can smile, smile, smile; in other words, it's the muscle you use to show you're happy. This "happy" muscle originates at the outer cheekbone and terminates in the skin and muscle which surrounds the mouth. When you are smiling, your cheeks must go up with the corners of your mouth — and we all know that what goes up isn't drooping down.

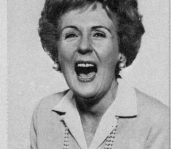

The Use:

IN EXPRESSIVE ACTION:
Riddle: Q: What disappears every time you stand up?
A: Your lap. (Did you laugh? If you did, you used your Zygomaticus, and *I'm* glad.)
Q: What disappears every time you laugh? A: A sad sack's sagging muscles. (Which should make *you* glad.)

44

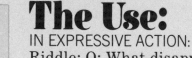

The Exercise:

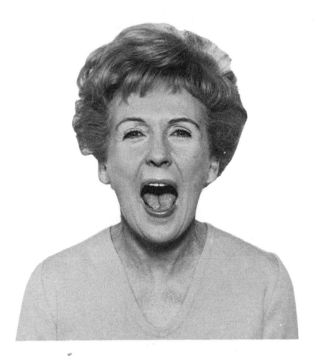

1. Make a great big open-mouthed smile. As you do so, try to make the corners of your mouth turn upward.

2. Now, try to make your upward smile bigger and bigger as you say the words, "Ha. Ha. Ha. Ha. Ha." Say them to yourself, or aloud—it doesn't matter. Bobbing your head a bit, however, as if you were really laughing, may help you exercise the "laughing" muscle just a little better.

DO EXERCISE **5** TIMES BEFORE RETURNING MOUTH TO NORMAL POSITION.

14 Raising a Furrow
TO DE-EMPHASIZE THE NOSE-TO-MOUTH FURROW

The Muscle:
The *Caninus* (kā nī' nus) and the Triangularis work together to pull the lips medialward. Working with two heads of the Quadratus labii superioris, the Caninus helps to create the furrows which outline the cheek and mouth area. The Caninus originates under cover of the Caput zygomaticum head of the Quadratus labii superioris. As it extends downward, the Caninus intermingles with muscles of the mouth and terminates in the skin at the medial line of the lower lip. A toned Caninus pulls the face up into an expression of gladness.

The Use:
IN EXPRESSIVE ACTION:
"Look at me, I'm holding a smile for the photographer." If you smile and hold it—as I am doing—you, too, will be using your Caninus.

46

The Exercise:

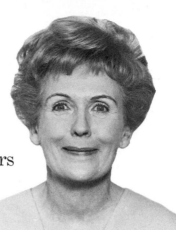

1. Smile with your lips together, turning corners of mouth in an upward direction.

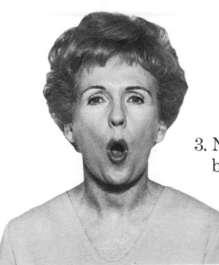

2. Keep smiling upward and separate your lips to make a "toothless" upward smile. In other words, cover your teeth with your lips.

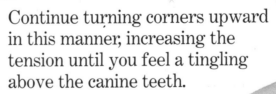

Continue turning corners upward in this manner; increasing the tension until you feel a tingling above the canine teeth.

3. Now, still keeping your teeth covered, slowly bring your mouth to an "O" shape.

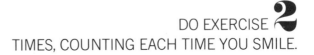

DO EXERCISE **2**
TIMES, COUNTING EACH TIME YOU SMILE.

15 The Teeth Clencher
TO HELP ALLEVIATE JOWLS; TO FIRM AND CONTOUR SIDES OF THE FACE

The Muscle:
The *Masseter* (ma sē' ter) closes the jaws, and when fully contracted, clenches the teeth, thus providing assistance to other muscles as food is chewed. The Masseter is a broad muscle, divided into two portions, one deep and the other superficial, and is situated at the sides of the face, extending from cheekbone to the lower jaw. Only a toned Masseter can counteract gravity's tendency to pull the jaw open. A jaw dropped by gravity is responsible for the be-jowled and flabby look at the sides of the face.

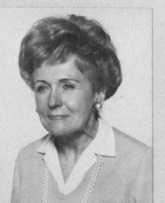

The Use:
IN EXPRESSIVE ACTION: "Grit your teeth and be determined." This action will best beat gravity at its open-jaw policy.

The Exercise:

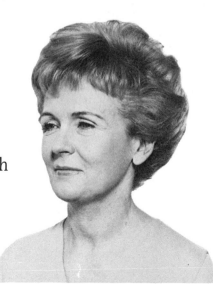

1. With mouth closed, clench the back teeth in a "dentist's bite."

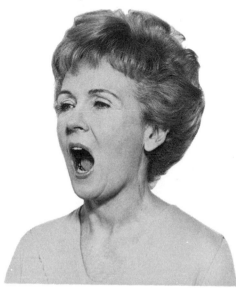

2. Release the clench and open the mouth.

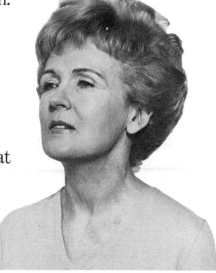

3. Slowly bring your lower jaw up so that the back molars meet again.

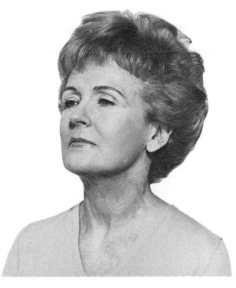

4. Now, bite down hard on these teeth.

DO EXERCISE **10** TIMES, COUNTING EACH TIME YOU BITE DOWN ON BACK MOLARS.

4th Day
Lower Cheek & Lips

It's an old wives' tale that what we are shows in our faces. This can be more than a tale if you don't use the lower cheek muscles enough to keep them in tone, or because of a mannerism, you use some of them so much they become literally fixed into a contraction.

How can you tell which type you are? If you have sunken cheeks, droopy lower cheeks, furrows between lower lip and chin that have gradually deepened, crepy skin around the lips, vertical wrinkles on the upper lip, pouches at mouth corners, smile lines around the mouth—it doesn't matter which type you are—you will need to do this group of exercises with regularity.

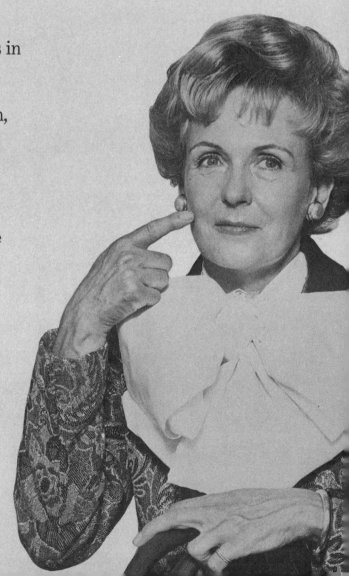

50

The 4th Day's Program

Pages 52-61

Do:

Exercise 1	The Scalp Raiser	20 times
Exercise 2	The Defrowner	5 times
Exercise 3	The Bridge Crosser	5 times
Exercise 4	The Eye Squeeze	5 times
Exercise 5	The Cryer	3 times
Exercise 6	The Eye Stretcher	3 times
Exercise 7	The Bag Trick	3 times
Exercise 8	The Eye Opener	3 times
Exercise 9	The Eye Resister	5 times
Exercise 10	The Nose Wrinkler	5 times
Exercise 11	The Cheek Raiser	5 times
Exercise 12	The Lid Lifter	5 times
Exercise 13	The Big Laugh	5 times
Exercise 14	Raising a Furrow	2 times
Exercise 15	The Teeth Clencher	10 times

New Exercises:

Exercise 16	The Slit of a Grin	5 times
Exercise 17	Miss Priss	5 times
Exercise 18	The Blotted Kiss	5 times
Exercise 19	The Upper-Lip Squeeze	5 times
Exercise 20	The Lower-Lip Squeeze	5 times

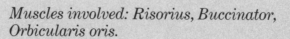

Muscles involved: Risorius, Buccinator, Orbicularis oris.

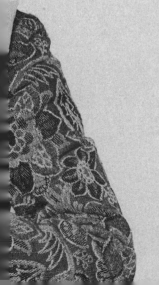

16 The Slit of a Grin
TO HELP ALLEVIATE POUCHES AT MOUTH CORNERS

The Muscle: The *Risorius* (ri sō′ ri us) draws the lips into a straight line toward the earlobes. It is a thin flat muscle that begins in the tissues of the Masseter and terminates in the skin at the corners of the mouth. A weak Risorius leaves a tell-tale sign on the face—pouches at mouth corners. A toned Risorius, in addition to alleviating these pouches, will contribute to firmness of cheeks.

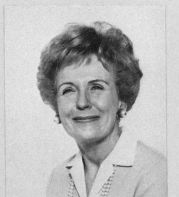

The Use:

IN EXPRESSIVE ACTION: The slit of a grin—often occasioned by an unfunny joke—brings the Risorius into use. Some describe the Risorius smile as "a way of saying Ugh! politely."

The Exercise:

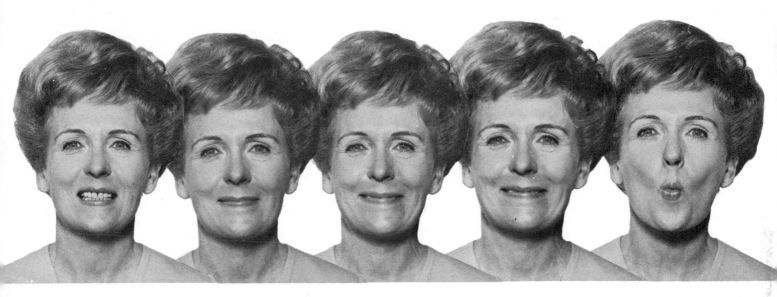

1. Put the edges of your teeth together. Hold them in this position throughout the exercise. Close your lips over your teeth.

2. Now, slowly move the corners of your mouth outward to make a slit of a grin. Make as wide a grin as you can without showing any teeth. All the pull should be felt at the corners of the mouth. Let the corners open slightly.

3. Still keeping teeth together, bring corners of the mouth in, to an exaggerated "puckered kiss" position.

DO EXERCISE **5** TIMES, COUNTING EACH TIME YOU GRIN.

17 Miss Priss

TO HELP FIRM LOWER-CHEEK AREA

The Muscle:
The *Buccinator* (buk′ sin ā tor) presses the cheeks inward, bringing them into contact with the teeth, as in sucking; helps to force air out between the lips, as in blowing a trumpet; and holds food under immediate pressure of the teeth while eating. The Buccinator is the principal muscle of the lower cheek and forms the side wall of the oral cavity. It is a broad muscle originating in the upper and lower jaw in the region of the molar teeth, its fibers extending to the mouth, where it joins with other muscles and the Orbicularis oris to form the lips.

The signs of a weak Buccinator: crepy, loose skin in the lower-cheek area.

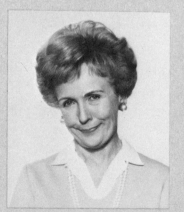

The Use:
IN EXPRESSIVE ACTION: Think: "You're silly!" This thought should make you draw your cheeks in toward your teeth, and thus use your Buccinator.

The Exercise:

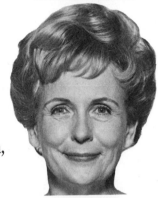

1. Put your lips together and smile slightly.

2. Holding your mouth in this position, suck the corners of your mouth in toward your teeth.

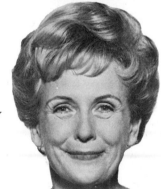

3. Keep the corners sucked in and try to pull the rest of your inner cheek in toward your teeth. Hold this contraction for the count of 10.

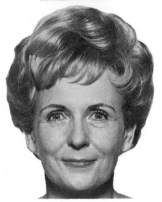

4. Slowly release suction, and then the smile.

DO EXERCISE **5** TIMES, COUNTING EACH TIME YOU SMILE.

18 The Blotted Kiss
TO BRING NATURAL COLOR TO THE LIPS AND TONE THE SURROUNDING SKIN

The Muscle:
The *Orbicularis oris* (or bik ū lā′ ris   ō′ ris) surrounds the opening of the mouth and helps to form the fleshy portion of the lips. Unlike the muscle surrounding the eye, it is not a simple sphincter muscle with a single functionary action. Its proper fibers close the mouth, but *how* the mouth is closed is determined by the degree of contraction and relaxation of the fibers it gains from a dozen other facial muscles. (As you will see in Exercises 19 and 20.)

Upwardly, the Orbicularis oris is limited by the nose; downwardly, by the junction of the lower lip and chin. By increasing the circulation to the fleshy portion of the lips, one can help keep the lips moist and soft as well as bring to them a more natural color.

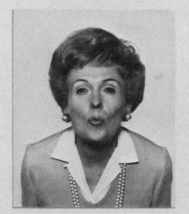

The Use:
IN EXPRESSIVE ACTION: Pucker your lips, making them protrude as far as you can. Does it look as if you are trying to kiss yourself? Good! Then you're using the right muscles.

The Exercise:

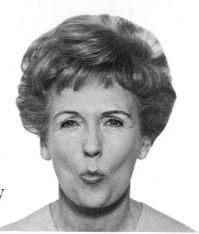

1. Bring mouth to a "kiss" position, with lips puckered together as tightly as possible.

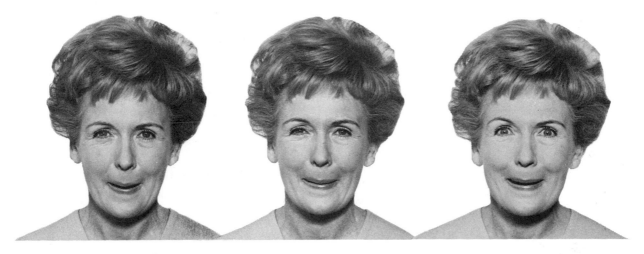

2. Now, slowly release the pucker. As you release it, open lips slightly and begin to turn them inward as some women do when they blot their lipstick.

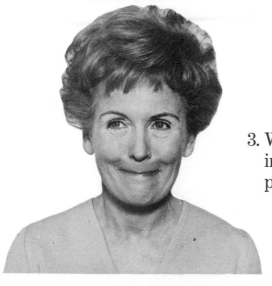

3. When lips are completely turned inward, close the mouth in this position, and press the lips together.

DO EXERCISE **5** TIMES, COUNTING EACH TIME YOU PUCKER LIPS.

57

19 The Upper-Lip Squeeze
TO HELP SMOOTH AND FIRM UPPER-LIP AREA

The Muscle: The *Orbicularis oris* in its ordinary action closes the lips. However, the mouth is contorted into various shapes by the degree of contraction of the muscles that blend and/or insert in the fibers of the Orbicularis oris and its surrounding skin. (See drawing.) It is these accessory muscles which, in the main, account for the tonus condition of the lip area.

One can't totally separate the action of the two lips and their accessory muscles, but to bring the upper-lip area more quickly into tonus condition, it is important to try — for in this manner, more fibers of the accessory muscles will be activated to make the required lip movements.

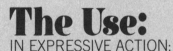

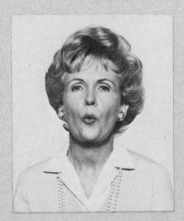

The Use:
IN EXPRESSIVE ACTION: Fellows whistle inwardly to show their appreciation of a girl who's passing by. Try it, girl or no girl, to get the accessory muscles of your upper lip working.

The Exercise:

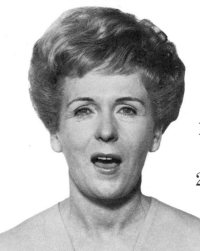

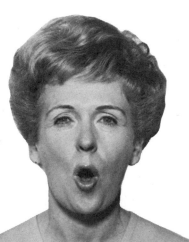

1. Lower your jaw to part lips slightly.

2. Hold this open position and pucker your lips.

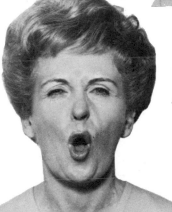

3. Bring more of a pucker to your upper lip by squeezing the nostrils of your nose together.

4. At the same time, try to keep the muscles in your lower lip as relaxed as possible.

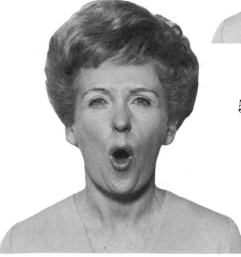

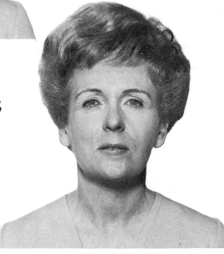

5. Slowly release pucker, returning mouth to natural position.

DO EXERCISE **5** TIMES, COUNTING EACH TIME YOU PUCKER UPPER LIP.

20 The Lower-Lip Squeeze

TO HELP LESSEN FURROWS FROM MOUTH CORNERS TO CHIN

The Muscle: As accessory
muscles to the *Orbicularis oris*, the
Quadratus labii inferioris and the
Mentalis function as movers of the
lower lip, along with the Buccinator,
Risorius, Triangularis, Caninus
and Platysma, which serve both
lips. The interaction—or lack of it
—between these lower-lip movers
is responsible for the furrows
deepening from the mouth corners
to the chin's edge. Endeavoring
the impossible—that is, trying to
move the lower lip without moving
the upper lip—will help to bring tone
to these lower-lip muscles more quickly.

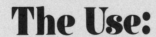

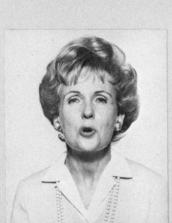

The Use:

IN EXPRESSIVE ACTION:
Open your mouth slightly and
stick your lower lip out a little.
How do you look? As if you were
saying, "Aah, I don't believe
it!"? That's the way you are apt
to look when you use the accessory muscles of the lower lip.

The Exercise:

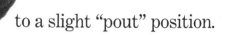

1. Lift lower lip up…   to a slight "pout" position.

2. Keep pout as much as you can and pucker the lower lip, as if you were trying to make its two corners meet in the center of the mouth.

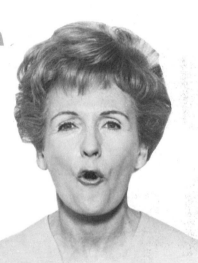

3. Slowly release pucker…   …to return mouth to natural position.

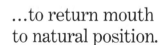

DO EXERCISE **5** TIMES, COUNTING EACH TIME YOU PUCKER LOWER LIP.

5th Day
Chin & Jawline

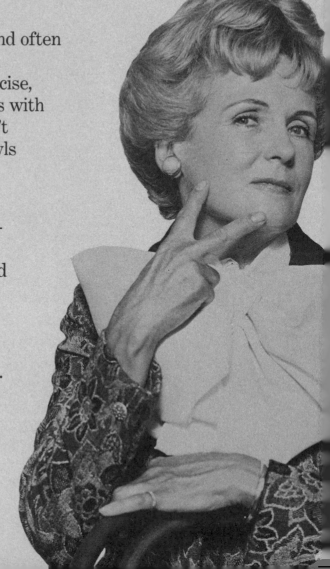

Even the thinnest person can develop jowls—and often does. Gravity pulls downward on facial muscles, so unless muscles are kept in tone through exercise, they will begin to sag. Men can cover their jowls with beards, but women aren't so fortunate. But don't despair; both men and women can get rid of jowls and other lower-chin problems by doing the next group of exercises—and two things more:

1. As you walk around all day, think about keeping the edges of your teeth together—and do it. Most of us let gravity separate our teeth instead of making muscles keep them together.

2. When riding in a car, when looking at TV— keep your mouth closed and bring your tongue up to touch your upper teeth and suck inwardly. Hold a little, release a while, then do it again…and again…

The 5th Day's Program
Pages 64-73

Do:

Exercise 1	The Scalp Raiser	*20 times*
Exercise 2	The Defrowner	*5 times*
Exercise 3	The Bridge Crosser	*5 times*
Exercise 4	The Eye Squeeze	*5 times*
Exercise 5	The Cryer	*3 times*
Exercise 6	The Eye Stretcher	*3 times*
Exercise 7	The Bag Trick	*3 times*
Exercise 8	The Eye Opener	*3 times*
Exercise 9	The Eye Resister	*5 times*
Exercise 10	The Nose Wrinkler	*5 times*
Exercise 11	The Cheek Raiser	*5 times*
Exercise 12	The Lid Lifter	*5 times*
Exercise 13	The Big Laugh	*5 times*
Exercise 14	Raising a Furrow	*2 times*
Exercise 15	The Teeth Clencher	*10 times*
Exercise 16	The Slit of a Grin	*5 times*
Exercise 17	Miss Priss	*5 times*
Exercise 18	The Blotted Kiss	*5 times*
Exercise 19	The Upper-Lip Squeeze	*5 times*
Exercise 20	The Lower-Lip Squeeze	*5 times*

New Exercises:

Exercise 21	The Big Chew	*20 times*
Exercise 22	The Stubborn Jaw	*6 times*
Exercise 23	The Chin Raiser	*5 times*
Exercise 24	A Show of Teeth	*5 times*
Exercise 25	Down at the Mouth	*5 times*

Muscles involved: Temporalis, Pterygoids, Mentalis, Quadratus labii inferioris, Triangularis.

21 The Big Chew

TO HELP ALLEVIATE DOUBLE CHIN

The Muscle: The *Temporalis* (tem po rā' lis) takes part in the movements of closing the jaw and clenching the teeth. In addition, it retracts the chin from a protruded position. It starts as a broad radiating muscle and converges as it descends, going under cover of the Masseter as it travels from the side of the head to its final termination in the lower jaw. When out of tone, the Temporalis contributes to the look of an underslung jaw, and to the making of a "double chin."

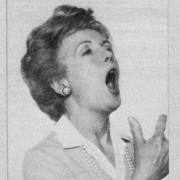

The Use:

IN EXPRESSIVE ACTION:
Open your mouth as wide as you can and sing out your top note. To do this, you will pull your chin back, thus activating your Temporalis. When you stop singing, and close your mouth, your Temporalis will help you do that, too.

64

The Exercise:

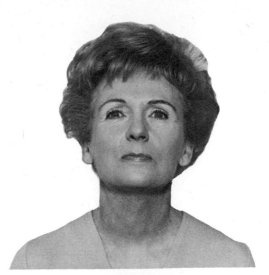

1. Hold your head upright throughout exercise, with chin tilted up slightly and lips firmly closed.

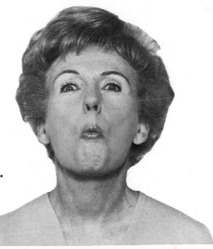

2. Slowly separate lower teeth from upper teeth, getting as much distance between them as you can without letting lips part...

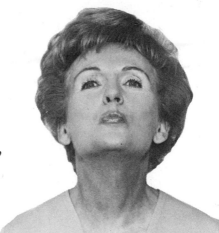

3. Slowly return teeth to normal position, to conclude one exaggerated "chewing" motion.

DO EXERCISE **20** TIMES, COUNTING EACH TIME YOU SEPARATE TEETH.

22 The Stubborn Jaw
TO HELP ALLEVIATE JOWLS AND DOUBLE CHIN

The Muscle:
The *Pterygoids* (ter' i goyds) are the muscles which, when properly used, help prevent the jaw from being underslung. There are two sets of Pterygoids, internal and external. The internal set closes the jaw and helps with the chewing action. The external set opens the jaw, protrudes it and moves it from side to side. The Pterygoids are partially exercised when the Masseter, the Digastric and Temporal muscles are used. The following exercise is designed to operate the fibers of the Pterygoids which have not previously been activated in an exercise, namely, those which help move the jaw forward and from side to side.

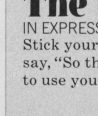

The Use:
IN EXPRESSIVE ACTION: Stick your jaw out and say, "So there," if you want to use your Pterygoids.

The Exercise:

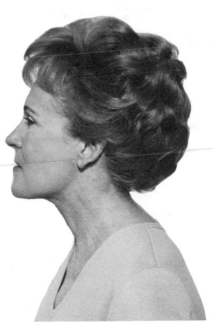

1. Keep lips together.
   Separate teeth slightly.

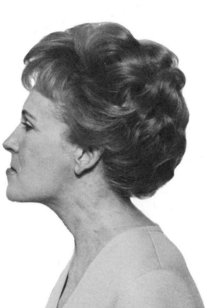

2. Push your lower jaw
   forward as far as you can, to
   "lead with your chin." Keeping
   chin forward, slowly move it
   from side to side 6 times.

3. Slowly bring jaw back
   to its starting position.

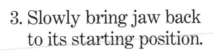

DO EXERCISE **10**
TIMES, COUNTING EACH TIME YOU "LEAD WITH YOUR CHIN."

23 The Chin Raiser
TO HELP FIRM AND SMOOTH THE SKIN OF THE CHIN

The Muscle:
The *Mentalis* (men tā′ lis) pushes the lower lip to a pout position and simultaneously raises the skin at the tip of the chin. The Mentali originate just below the incisor teeth on the right and left sides of the lower jaw. They terminate in the skin near the tip of the chin where the fibers of the two Mentali often intermingle at the medial line. The Mentalis is the skin mover of the central portion of the chin. If you've got chin problems, the Mentalis can smooth them out for you.

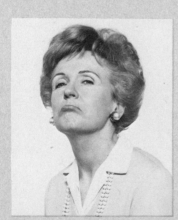

The Use:
IN EXPRESSIVE ACTION: To show disappointment, some people have been known to use their Mentalis—that is, they have pushed up their under lip and pouted. Who—me? I'm not pouting—only demonstrating.

The Exercise:

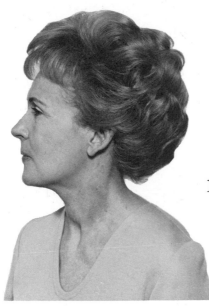

1. Close mouth, with lips relaxed.

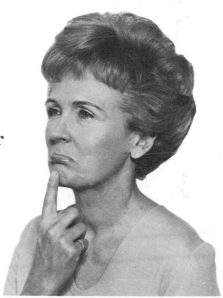

2. Use your chin muscle to push your lower lip up into a "pout" position. (The muscle to be used is indicated by my finger.)

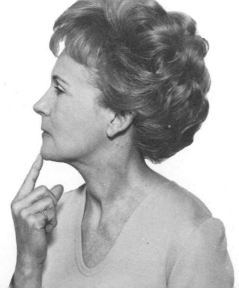

3. Now, slowly pull chin back to starting position.

(Those with a "double chin" problem should keep face parallel to the ceiling while doing this exercise.)

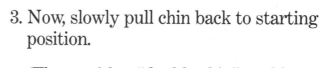

DO EXERCISE **5** TIMES, COUNTING EACH TIME YOU PUSH CHIN UP.

24 A Show of Teeth

TO HELP SMOOTH THE SKIN AT THE CORNERS OF THE MOUTH AND UPPER CHIN

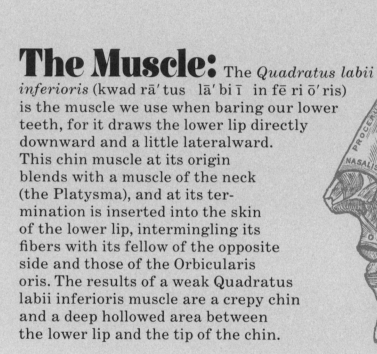

The Muscle:

The *Quadratus labii inferioris* (kwad rā′tus lā′bi ī in fē ri ō′ris) is the muscle we use when baring our lower teeth, for it draws the lower lip directly downward and a little lateralward. This chin muscle at its origin blends with a muscle of the neck (the Platysma), and at its termination is inserted into the skin of the lower lip, intermingling its fibers with its fellow of the opposite side and those of the Orbicularis oris. The results of a weak Quadratus labii inferioris muscle are a crepy chin and a deep hollowed area between the lower lip and the tip of the chin.

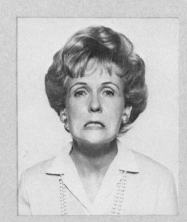

The Use:

IN EXPRESSIVE ACTION:
Bare your teeth in mock anger as if you were growling back at a dog, and you will have used your Quadratus labii inferioris.

The Exercise:

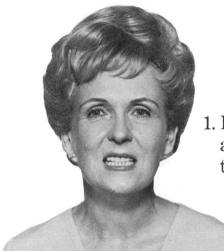

1. Look directly into the mirror and place the edges of your teeth together.

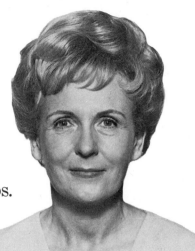

2. Close lips.

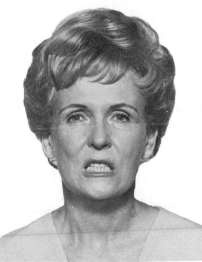

3. Keeping teeth together, slowly pull lower lip downward. Pull it downward as far as you can. (When done correctly, the lower lip will curl over slightly in the center and you will see the inside of the lower lip.)

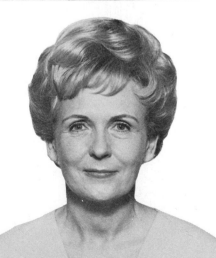

4. Slowly return lip to normal position.

DO EXERCISE **5** TIMES, COUNTING EACH TIME YOU PULL LIP DOWN.

25 Down at the Mouth
TO HELP LESSEN FURROWS FROM MOUTH CORNERS TO CHIN

The Muscle: The *Triangularis*
(trī ang gū lā′ ris) turns the corners of the mouth downward, and in addition, with help from the Caninus, draws the corners of the mouth toward one another. This triangular-shaped muscle originates at the chin line. Its fibers extend upward, converging at the corners of the lips, where they blend, attach and insert into other muscles of the mouth.

The action of the Triangularis contributes a sad expression to the face; its inaction can contribute furrows and pouches from the lower lip down — and what could be sadder than that!

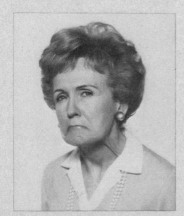

The Use:
IN EXPRESSIVE ACTION:
Turn the corners of your mouth downward, emulating the lines cartoonists and clowns use to create a look of anguished sadness — and you will have used your Triangularis. Are you sad? You will look it — but I hope only for a minute.

The Exercise:

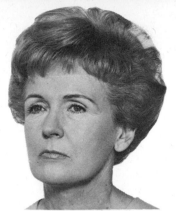

1. Bring your lips to a pursed position.

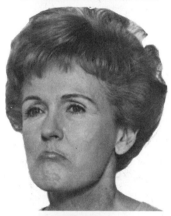

2. Use the muscle at the tip of your chin to push "pursed" lips upward. When lips are pushed up as far as they will go...

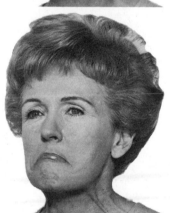

3. ...hold the upward tension with your chin and pull the corners of your mouth downward. Hold downward contraction for the count of 5.

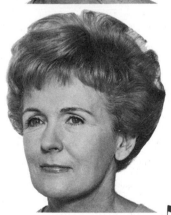

4. Then slowly return lips to horizontal position.

DO EXERCISE **5**
TIMES, COUNTING EACH TIME YOU PUSH LIPS UPWARD.

6th Day
Under-Chin & Throat

There are many causes of a "double chin." My experience indicates that the common causes are: 1. A constantly relaxed lower jaw. 2. Weak chewing muscles. 3. Weakened jaw-opening muscles. 4. Excess weight. 5. Improper head carriage. 6. Poor sitting and standing posture.

The exercises which follow will be particularly helpful to those with double chins caused by items 1 through 3. They will be helpful to a limited extent for double chins caused by items 4 through 6. Those who have double chins due to excess weight, in addition to doing the exercises, will need to diet. Those whose head carriage or posture is a contributing factor to their double chins will need to do these exercises, and in addition, strengthen posture muscles with exercises such as I recommend in my *21-Day Shape-Up Program.** As the under-chin muscles are strengthened, the throat and neck-area muscles will also be brought into tone.

Published by Random House, 1968.

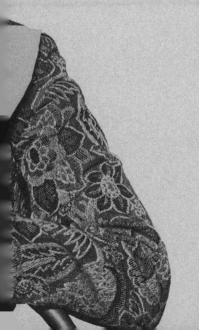

The 6th Day's Program
Pages 76-85

Do:

Exercise 1	*The Scalp Raiser*	*20 times*
Exercise 2	*The Defrowner*	*5 times*
Exercise 3	*The Bridge Crosser*	*5 times*
Exercise 4	*The Eye Squeeze*	*5 times*
Exercise 5	*The Cryer*	*3 times*
Exercise 6	*The Eye Stretcher*	*3 times*
Exercise 7	*The Bag Trick*	*3 times*
Exercise 8	*The Eye Opener*	*3 times*
Exercise 9	*The Eye Resister*	*5 times*
Exercise 10	*The Nose Wrinkler*	*5 times*
Exercise 11	*The Cheek Raiser*	*5 times*
Exercise 12	*The Lid Lifter*	*5 times*
Exercise 13	*The Big Laugh*	*5 times*
Exercise 14	*Raising a Furrow*	*2 times*
Exercise 15	*The Teeth Clencher*	*10 times*
Exercise 16	*The Slit of a Grin*	*5 times*
Exercise 17	*Miss Priss*	*5 times*
Exercise 18	*The Blotted Kiss*	*5 times*
Exercise 19	*The Upper-Lip Squeeze*	*5 times*
Exercise 20	*The Lower-Lip Squeeze*	*5 times*
Exercise 21	*The Big Chew*	*20 times*
Exercise 22	*The Stubborn Jaw*	*6 times*
Exercise 23	*The Chin Raiser*	*5 times*
Exercise 24	*A Show of Teeth*	*5 times*
Exercise 25	*Down at the Mouth*	*5 times*

New Exercises:

Exercise 26	*The Gaper*	*10 times*
Exercise 27	*The Head Raiser*	*10 times*
Exercise 28	*The Tongue Depressor*	*5 times*
Exercise 29	*"Ceiling" a Kiss*	*5 times*
Exercise 30	*Stiff-Necked*	*5 times*

Muscles involved: Digastricus, Sternocleido-mastoideus, Mylohyoideus, Platysma, All neck muscles.

75

26 The Gaper
TO HELP ALLEVIATE DOUBLE CHIN

The Muscle:
The *Digastricus* (dī gas' tri kus) assists in opening the jaws. It has two fleshy parts, one longer than the other, which are united in the neck by a tendon. The longer part of the muscle arises from behind the ear; the shorter, from a depression in the chin bone. The two parts meet under the chin to form a sling-like muscle, and are attached by a tendon to the hyoid bone. The anterior (shorter) portion of the muscle draws this neck bone forward. The posterior (longer) portion draws it backward. This two-part Digastric muscle—rarely put to full use because gravity does most of the mouth-opening job—can help determine whether you have a one- or two-part chin.

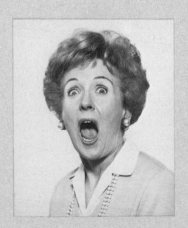

The Use:
IN EXPRESSIVE ACTION: Open-mouthed wonder? No wonder! You must have used the Digastric muscle.

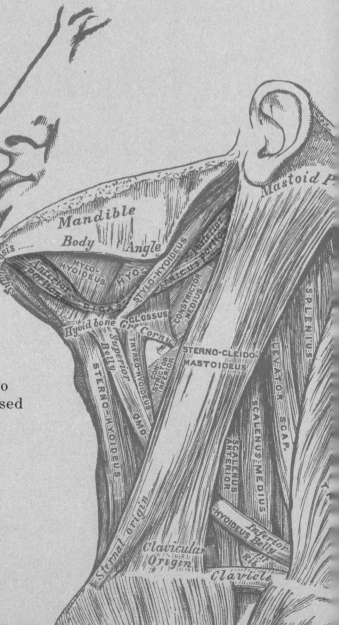

The Exercise:

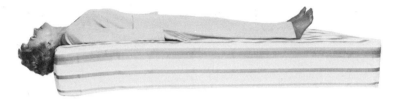

1. Lie down on a bed with your head hanging over the edge.

2. Slowly open your mouth.

3. Slowly close your mouth.

DO EXERCISE **10** TIMES, COUNTING EACH TIME YOU OPEN JAWS.

27 The Head Raiser

TO HELP ALLEVIATE A CREPY NECK BY LENGTHENING NECK

The Muscle:

The *Sternocleido-mastoideus* (ster nō klī′ do mas toyd′ ē us) turns the head from side to side; brings it toward the shoulder; thrusts the head forward; tilts it backward, elevating the chin as it does so, and in addition, helps to hold the head upright. It is literally the "outstanding" muscle of the neck, and a turn of your head to one side will prove it. The Sternocleidomastoid muscle is the thickest and strongest muscle at the side of the neck. It extends upward from the breast and collarbone along the side of the neck to terminate in the temporal bone behind the ear.

Neck wrinkles occur when the Sternocleidomastoideus is out of tone and fails to keep the neck in a stretched upward position.

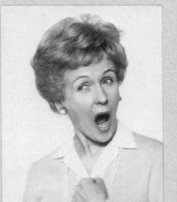

The Use:

IN EXPRESSIVE ACTION: Turn your head and say, "I'm as smart as you are," and you'll use your Sternocleidomastoideus. (See that big muscle sticking out on my neck?)

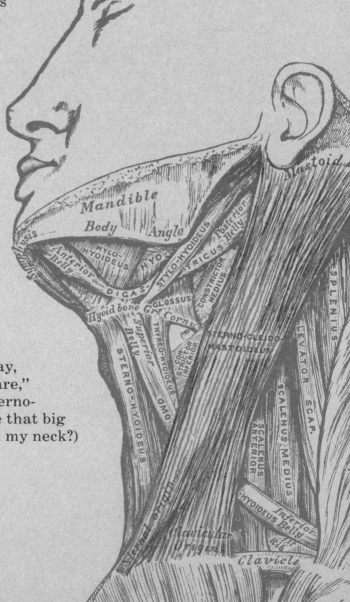

78

The Exercise:

1. Lie down on a bed with your head hanging over the edge.

2. Slowly raise your head so that it is level with your body.

3. Slowly lower head back down.

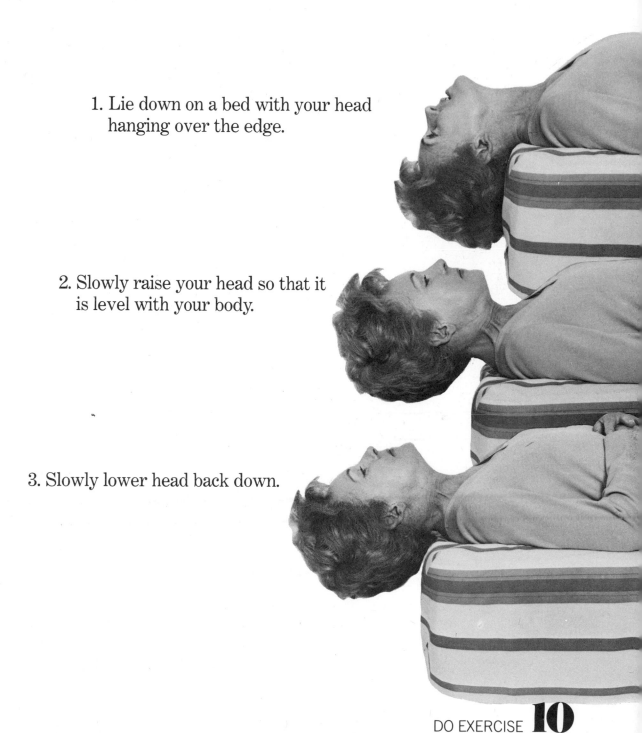

DO EXERCISE **10**
TIMES, COUNTING EACH TIME YOU RAISE HEAD.

28 The Tongue Depressor
TO HELP ALLEVIATE DOUBLE CHIN

The Muscle: The *Mylohyoideus*
(mī lō hī oyd′ ē us) raises the back of the tongue
and the hyoid bone (a motion essential to the
act of swallowing). It is a flat triangular
muscle, which, with its fellow of the
opposite side, forms a muscular floor
for the cavity of the mouth. Because
of its attachment to the hyoid bone
(situated at the middle of the neck),
this muscle helps determine the outward appearance of the under-chin area.

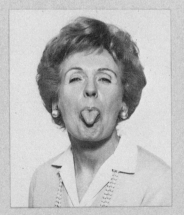

The Use:
IN EXPRESSIVE ACTION:
Stick out your tongue to
show your displeasure—and you
will have used your Mylohyoideus
muscle to do it.

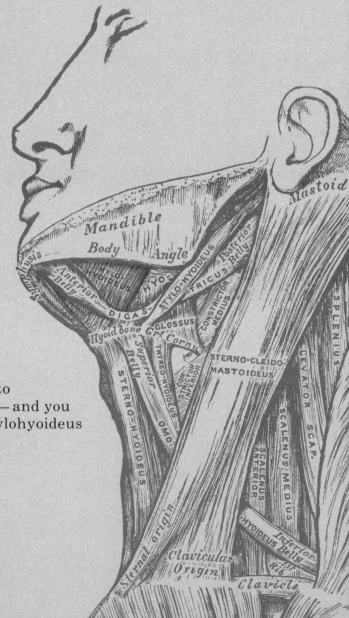

The Exercise:

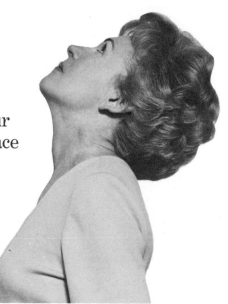

1. Assume a standing position. Put your head back on your shoulders, with face parallel to the ceiling.

2. Stick your tongue out in a downward direction as far as it will go.

3. Return tongue to mouth. Return head to normal position.

DO EXERCISE **5** TIMES, COUNTING EACH TIME YOU STICK OUT TONGUE.

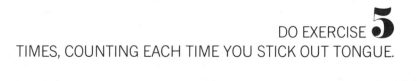

81

29 "Ceiling" a Kiss
TO HELP SMOOTH THE SKIN OF THE NECK

The Muscle: The *Platysma*
(plah tiz' mah) controls the skin at the side
of the neck. It pulls it upward from the
collarbone region of the chest to increase the
neck diameter and release the pressure of
a tight collar. It draws the lower lip downward to widen the aperture at the corners
of the mouth. These are not particularly attractive actions, but must be
done if the Platysma is to be toned.
The Platysma is a broad thin sheet
of muscle which extends upward
from the chest area to the jaw and
chin region of the face. When in
tone, the Platysma acts as the smooth
cover for the more active neck muscles
and thus alleviates the crepy-neck look.

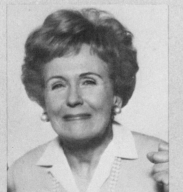

The Use:
IN EXPRESSIVE ACTION:
Act out, as if you meant
it, the phrase, "I was so mad
I busted a collar button," and
you will have used all the
fibers of the Platysma,
"that old smoothie."

82

The Exercise:

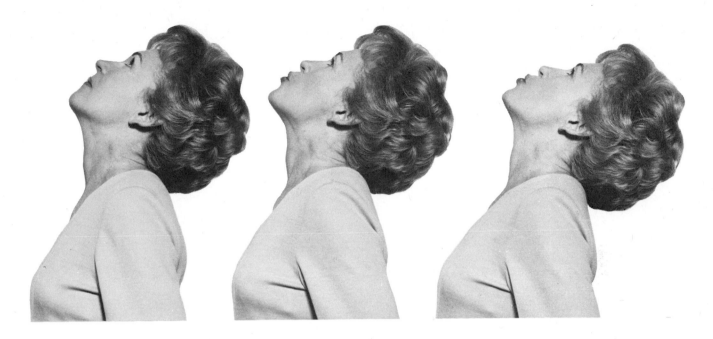

1. Drop head back on shoulders so face is parallel to the ceiling.

2. Bring lips to a "puckered kiss" position.

3. Exaggerate the "kiss" position as you maintain head position. Stretch that kiss up as if you were trying to kiss the ceiling. Keep stretching until you feel a tingling sensation.

4. Slowly release the pucker. Grin widely at the ceiling. Pull corners of your mouth downward.

DO EXERCISE **5** TIMES, COUNTING EACH TIME YOU "KISS" CEILING.

The Muscle:

The muscles of the neck act together in multiple ways. None acts alone; some act together to bring the head backward, others bring it forward, some bend it to the side; the very same ones acting together can rotate the head. The neck muscles' interactions are complicated to explain, but easy to move. It's necessary to move them, too, unless you want them to quickly show "their" age.

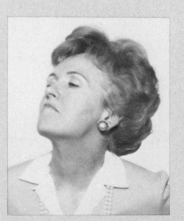

The Use:

IN EXPRESSIVE ACTION: Ever feel "like sticking your neck way out"? Well, do it, and you'll be loosening up a half dozen or more neck muscles. Who said it didn't pay to stick your neck out?

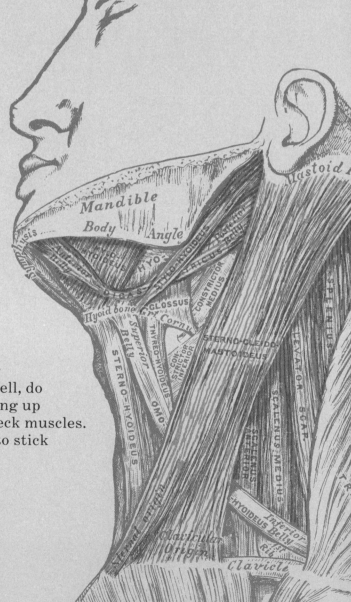

The Exercise:

1. Drop head back onto shoulders so that face is parallel to the ceiling. The further back you get your head, the better stretch you'll get.

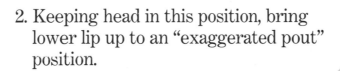

2. Keeping head in this position, bring lower lip up to an "exaggerated pout" position.

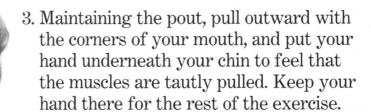

3. Maintaining the pout, pull outward with the corners of your mouth, and put your hand underneath your chin to feel that the muscles are tautly pulled. Keep your hand there for the rest of the exercise.

4. Now, return head to normal position. As you do so, move the head in such a way that the muscles under the chin remain taut.

DO EXERCISE **5** TIMES, COUNTING EACH TIME HEAD IS PARALLEL TO CEILING.

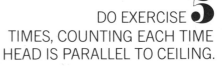

85

Index

All figures refer to page numbers except where otherwise noted:

Pterygoids, 22; Temporalis, 21
Dimpled hollows in cheekbone area?
Buccinator, 17; Caput zygo-
maticum, 12; Zygomaticus, 13

Chin and Jawline
Crepy chin?
Buccinator, 17; Mentalis, 23;
Orbicularis oris, 18, 19, 20;
Platysma, 29; Quadratus labii
inferioris, 24; Risorius, 16;
Triangularis, 25
Hollowed area beneath lower lip?
Caninus, 14; Platysma, 29;
Quadratus labii inferioris, 24;
Risorius, 16; Triangularis, 25
Jowls?
Digastricus, 26; Masseter, 15;
Mylohyoideus, 28; Platysma, 29;
Pterygoids, 22; Temporalis, 21
Furrows from mouth corners to
jawline?
Buccinator, 17; Mentalis, 23;
Quadratus labii inferioris, 24;
Triangularis, 25

Eyelids
Crepy, droopy, puffy upper eyelids?
Corrugator, 2; Frontalis, 1, 3;
Levator palpebrae, 8; Orbicularis
oculi, 4, 6, 7, 9; Tensor tarsi, 5
Crow's-feet?
Caput zygomaticum, 12; Frontalis,
1; Masseter, 15; Orbicularis
oculi, 4, 6, 7, 9; Temporalis, 21;
Zygomaticus, 13
Hollow circles under eyes?
Caput angulare, 10; Caput infra-
orbitale, 11; Caput zygomaticum,
12; Orbicularis oculi, 4, 7, 9;
Tensor tarsi, 5
Puffiness under eyes?
Caninus, 14; Caput angulare, 10;
Caput infra-orbitale, 11; Caput
zygomaticum, 12; Orbicularis oculi,
4, 7, 9; Tensor tarsi, 5;
Zygomaticus, 13
Squint lines under eyes?
Caninus, 14; Caput angulare, 10;
Caput infra-orbitale, 11; Caput
zygomaticum, 12; Orbicularis
oculi, 4, 7, 9; Zygomaticus, 13

Forehead and Scalp
Lines across forehead?
Corrugator 2; Frontalis, 1;
Procerus, 3
Frown lines between brows?
Corrugator 2; Frontalis, 1;
Sag between brows?
Frontalis 1; Procerus, 3

Nose
Lines and wrinkles at bridge of nose?
Caput angulare, 10; Corrugator, 2;
Frontalis, 1; Orbicularis oculi, 4,
6, 9; Procerus, 3
Sunburst of wrinkles between bridge
of nose and nostrils?
Caput angulare, 10; Frontalis, 1, 2, 3
Deep grooves at nose wings?
Caninus, 14; Caput angulare, 10

Upper Lip and Mouth
Vertical lines on upper lip?
Buccinator, 17; Caninus, 14; Caput
angulare, 10; Caput infra-orbitale,
11; Caput zygomaticum, 12;
Orbicularis oris, 18, 19, 20;
Risorius, 16; Zygomaticus, 13
Pouches at corners of upper lip?
Buccinator, 17; Caninus, 14;
Orbicularis oris, 18, 19, 20; Risorius,
16; Triangularis, 25; Zygomaticus, 13
Smile lines at sides of mouth?
Orbicularis oris, 18, 19, 20;
Platysma, 29; Quadratus labii
inferioris, 24; Risorius, 16;
Triangularis, 25

Under-Chin and Throat
Double chin?
All neck muscles, 30; Digastricus,
26; Masseter, 15; Mentalis, 23;
Mylohyoideus, 28; Platysma, 29;
Pterygoids, 22; Sternocleidomas-
toideus, 27; Temporalis, 21;
Triangularis, 25
Crepy neck?
All neck muscles, 26, 28, 30;
Platysma, 29; Sternocleidomas-
toideus, 27; Triangularis, 25
Thick neck?
All neck muscles, 26, 28, 30;
Platysma, 29; Sternocleidomas-
toideus, 27; Triangularis, 25

ABOUT THE AUTHOR: Marjorie Craig was born in Bangor, Maine, in the year 1912, a date that would seem to be belied by her youthful face and figure which make her her own best ad for the exercises she invented, adapted and tested over a period of thirty-five years to meet the needs of her thousands of private pupils. In 1968 she presented her exercises to the public in a book, *Miss Craig's 21-Day Shape-Up Program for Men & Women;* it became a best seller which remained at the top of the best-seller list for thirty-two weeks.

For the past eighteen years, Miss Craig has been the supervisor and teacher of exercises at Elizabeth Arden's New York Salon. Miss Craig developed her interest in physical education in early childhood. At seventeen, she persuaded her parents to send her to Arnold College (now Bridgeport University), where she received a B.S. in physical education, and then went on to take a postgraduate course in physical therapy at Columbia University Medical School. Upon finishing her courses, she was recruited by the Neurological Institute of the Columbia Presbyterian Medical Center, where she had had some of her in-service training, and spent the next seven years aiding men, women and children to rehabilitate muscles which they had damaged in accidents, or lost temporary use of through illness or surgery. She left the medical center to head the exercise program of Richard Hudnut's Fifth Avenue Salon, and remained there until the late Elizabeth Arden personally hired her away.

Miss Craig is Mrs. John T. Crowley in private life. The Crowleys have been married for thirty-five years; they live with their golden retriever, Sunny, in Bedford Village, New York.

She's using her...

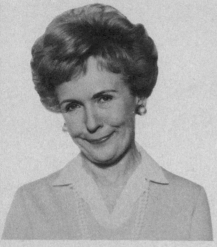
Buccinator

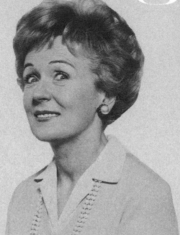
Caninus

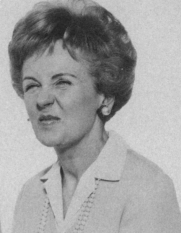
Caput angulare

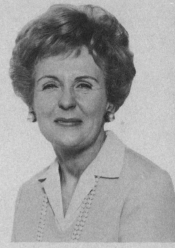
Caput infra-orbitale

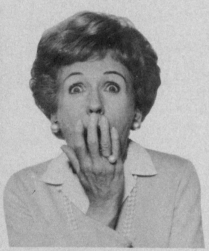
Levator palpebrae superioris

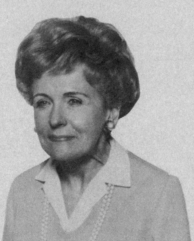
Masseter

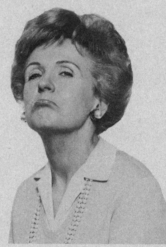
Mentalis

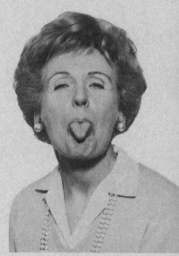
Mylohyoideus

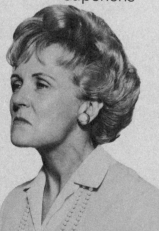
Pterygoids

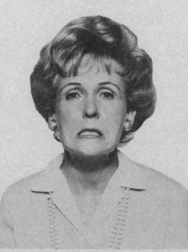
Quadratus labii inferioris

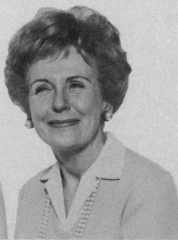
Risorius

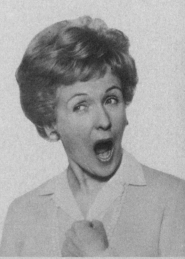
Sternocleidomastoideus